Medical Marijuana Guide

A Complete Guide for Understanding and Using Cannabis Medical Power. How to Relieve Chronic Pain, Anxiety, Insomnia and Depression with THC and CBD

BY

MATTHEW CAMPBELL

Table of Contents

INTRODUCTION

The fact that cannabis is useful in medicine is something of an open secret. It is a common knowledge that cannabis growers, bud lovers and medical practitioners share. The medical uses of the plant can be traced back to its origination itself. Man has for a long time used cannabis to cure many ailments. In recent times, medicinal cannabis has attracted a lot of attention that has unavoidably led to controversies relating to its legal, ethical and societal implications. People are continually worried about whether the use of cannabis is safe and would not result in further complications.

Medicinal cannabis is a specific treatment routine that lends itself to these complexities because of the limited clinical data available. Cannabis, otherwise known as marijuana, is a plant that is botanically active with substances that have found some usefulness in medicine. These substances can be found all over the plant, from its leaves to its buds and in its extracts. If grown properly, cannabis has a lot of chemical components that have become the subject of medical research and from which different medicines have been derived. These medicines have continued to be used for different purposes. Medical cannabis is great for treating a lot of symptoms and clinical conditions that we would explore in this book.

Medical authorities also see the plant as capable of being abused and used as an illicit drug. This reputation that cannabis has is a pivotal reason for its inability to get necessary medical approval despite that an entire treatment procedure hinges on it. The controversies surrounding cannabis and its use in medical treatments are juxtaposed with its continual acceptance in social situations.

It is important for anyone who is interested in cannabis to know what medical benefits the plant holds for him. In this book, we will explore how cannabis interacts with different ailments and symptoms of disease conditions to make them better. Medical cannabis has to do with the interplay between cannabis and the development of medicine. In certain instances such as pain, cannabis can provide instant relief. Why is it able to do that? This is a pivotal question that we would answer in this book.

If you have wondered how cannabis can be used to make a health situation better, then this book is for you. Knowing the right instances within which to use cannabis can keep you from making the wrong decisions. You will find that the chemical components of cannabis play a very important role in determining its medical viability. To help you gain a wider knowledge of the subject, we will examine how these components interact throughout this book.

This book will expose you to the specific uses of cannabis in medicine. At the end of the book, you would understand what the correct uses for cannabis are in clinical procedure, and what uses should be avoided. If this is an area you have been looking to explore, you should dig into the book already. Cannabis may be doing more for you than you know. Similarly, there are more potent use for cannabis than you realize. Let's explore medical marijuana together in the pages that follow.

CHAPTER ONE

GET TO KNOW YOUR CANNABIS

We cannot delve into medicinal marijuana without first taking an overall look at cannabis, its cultivation, its evolvement and the importance that it holds as a plant. Cannabis is popular for both its medicinal effects and its recreational usefulness. People call the plant different things like weed, herb, grass, pot, ganja, and so on. It comes with a certain relief that is almost heavenly. If you want a mental high or a body high, there is absolutely a cannabis strain that suits your ambition. There are several kinds of cannabis with each type having a particular purpose.

Regardless of what you need cannabis for; they are grouped into two broad strains. These are the indica and sativa strains. Medical cannabis also comes within these classes. Before we get into the details of medical marijuana, it would be helpful to understand these cannabis strains and their individual characteristics. Aside the indica and sativa strain, there is also a third cannabis strain called the hybrid strain. Hybrid cannabis are a combination of indica and sativa and are numerous. However, there is the Ruderalis strain that stands out of the flock. The Ruderalis strain is also called the auto-flowering strain. Each cannabis strain has a characteristic effect associated with it, and similar genetics within its family. Cannabis with the same genetics have been grouped into the same family. They possess similar traits that make it easy to determine the outcome of your final product by just choosing a suitable strain.

Despite the careful grouping, there are hybrid strains that are neither indica nor sativa in their characteristics. They have developed into a cannabis species of their own. The hybrid cannabis, Haze, comes within this category. In most cases, Hazes are on their own without lending to the characteristics of either family from which they originated. Sometimes however, they could be sativa or indica. Before we get into an exposition on the subject of medical cannabis, it is important for us to understand what these cannabis strains are and what growers look for when making cannabis.

Indica

Indica cannabis have rounder leaves than their sativa counterpart. Sativas are thinner. This cannabis strain grows bushy and is shorter than sativa. When you get a physical sensation that runs through your body from your cannabis, you are taking the indica strain. This cannabis gives you a high sensation all over your body.

Sativa

With the sativa strain of cannabis, you get a brain boost. This cannabis causes a mental high. A lot of people favor this cannabis strain over the indica strain. This cannabis strain grows larger and enjoys a robust growth. While growing sativa, there is the need for more than lighting to enable it grow to its full capacity. Sativas mature much later than indicas. As a result, the timeframe for its growth is much longer than the indica.

Hybrid

The hybrid strains of cannabis are popular because they give both a mental and a physical high. Also, they are easier to grow. In fact, the grower can decide to make cannabis strains of his choice. All he needs to do is get seeds or clones that have the characteristics that he wants in the final cannabis plant. He can also decide if he wants the new plant to be more indica or sativa. Hybrid strains are preferred by most people because they carry the best traits of both the sativa and the indica.

A good example of the hybrid strain is the ruderalis strain which has the ability to trigger flowering on its own regardless of the lighting conditions in which it is grown. No matter what happens with the light schedule around the auto-flowering strain, it would induce its own vegetative growth and make it to harvest.

BASICS OF GROWING CANNABIS

The hybrid cannabis strain exposes us to the fact of the farmer being able to determine beforehand what he wants to see in his cannabis plant. It becomes important to know precisely what he plants. Can hybrid cannabis be made out of seeds? And if they can, what should the grower look out for in his seeds? In this section, we will be looking at the important aspects of growing cannabis.

Seeds

This is the most natural way to begin a cannabis farm. In fact, they are the first things that come to mind when you want to grow anything at all. Perhaps, the reason why seeds are most often used is the fact that they are easy to get. It is possible to get your cannabis on the internet, and have them delivered to you. Also, it doesn't really matter where the seeds come from, they can be gotten from and taken to any part of the world.

Healthy and viable seeds are hard and dark colored. If the seeds are small and white, they will not germinate and any efforts put into growing them would have been in vain. Healthy seeds can be stored in a refrigerator but you must not allow them to freeze as this can spoil the seeds. Seeds are better kept dry and away from light. Growers often come across bagseeds when they purchase cannabis. These seeds are found mingled with their marijuana. You may even find such seeds in your medical cannabis. These seeds can be planted without any further precautionary methods set in place. However, the grower may find that many of the seeds are useless because of their gender that makes them unable to produce buds. When growing with seeds, the farmer does not know what to expect and cannot guarantee the traits that the seeds carry.

Some growers have found bagseeds useful but this can so easily be hinged on a matter of luck. They can be tricky because it is possible for them to be totally different from the marijuana in which they were found. But a grower can only know that in the end. There are trusted sources on the internet that sell cannabis seeds to people who want to grow them. Similarly, for people looking to use bagseeds for growing cannabis, they have to get their marijuana from trusted suppliers. Growing with seeds is a popular method because they are easy to get and can set you up quickly. A little research is enough to set the process of getting the seeds and growing it in motion.

Clones

Cannabis can be grown using clones. Clones are exact copies of cannabis plants. The great thing about the cloning method for growing cannabis is that the grower can determine the traits of the final plant from the start. All he has to do is choose a mother plant that has the characteristics that he wants in the final plant. The clone will produce similar buds like those of the mother plant. This method is great because the grower can predict the traits of the cannabis that is produced. He also knows what kind of yield to expect.

A grower that intends to use this method must find a mother plant that he wants to clone. Unlike seeds that can be gotten online, clones are not easy to get on a regular basis. For people who are growing cannabis for medical purposes, clones may come easier to get. With a doctor's recommendation, you can get cannabis from your local medical marijuana dispensary.

Cannabis clones have to stay moist and be properly looked after until they grow roots. While light is important to growing cannabis, clones do not need as much lighting. They need warmth that fluorescent tubes are enough to provide. The clones get water from their leaves to sustain them until their roots begin to form. As a result, the leaves must remain moist. Automatic cloners already come with heat settings that regulate the temperature and keep it within the desired range.

Effective Cannabis Growing Conditions

Once the farmer has made the decision on whether he intends to use a seed or a clone, he has to determine also which growing methods will work for him. He also has to get the necessary tools in place. He can choose between outdoor growing and indoor growing. Although each method has its advantages and disadvantages, they lend to a different level of energy. This is mostly because the indoor growing method of cannabis has to do with replicating the growing techniques applicable outdoors and the conditions that enable them in a more controlled environment. While growing cannabis outdoors, the natural growing elements would work to enhance growth. For indoor growers, they have to set these elements in motion to achieve similar results. We will do a brief exposition of the conditions that enable cannabis growth in this section.

Feminized Seeds

Cannabis plants come in male and female. You would not be able to know the gender of your cannabis plants while they are still seeds. When it is time for harvest however, it is easy to determine the gender of a cannabis plant. For clones, you can determine their gender from the onset because they adopt the gender of the parent plant. A cannabis clone will give you the exact replica of the parent plant. Determining the parent plant is all up to you including the traits, genetics and gender. While female cannabis produce buds, male cannabis produce pollens. The pollen can cause seed production and pollination, and can inhibit the growth of the buds. You need the buds for your marijuana. This makes the male plants useless in most growing instances except during sexing. Growers often throw the male seeds away on sight. When you have all female seeds ready for planting, it is said that you have feminized seeds. These are what you should look out for when growing cannabis. They produce the buds needed for marijuana of all kinds.

Cannabis Life Cycle

Cannabis undergoes two stages of growth which are the vegetative stage and the flowering stage. The life cycle of cannabis lasts three to four months within which they would have completed their stages of growth. During the vegetative stage, cannabis propels all its energy into becoming a full grown, healthy and viable plant. At the flowering stage, it then produces the buds that are needed for marijuana. The plant is so sensitive that its growth is influenced by nature and time fluctuations in form of day and night. While cannabis love to rest, they love to get a lot of light too. During longer days, they enjoy a robust growth and the plant turns out big. The cannabis plants move from seed to seedling, vegetation and then to flowering. After the flowering stage, growers can now harvest their buds.

At the vegetative stage, the plant directs its energy into growing its support system which is its roots and stems, and its leaves. At the flowering stage, cannabis grows flowers and buds. When these are mature, the grower can move on to harvest. The vegetative stage begins at early spring and takes the plant all the way to summer. With outdoor growing, all these processes are set in motion naturally. With indoor growing however, the farmer has to create the right conditions to enable them occur. Usually, grow lights can give the plant the illusion of day and night if they are set correctly. The grow lights will give the plant an indication of when each season has started. Growers often use a timer to determine the growing period and to regulate lighting accordingly. The timer can also ignite each stage of growth in the plant.

Lighting

Lighting is essential to growing cannabis. Your plants need light, whether that light is natural or artificial. For people who grow cannabis indoors, they induce the proper level of lighting in their grow area through artificial lights called grow lights. Natural light on the other hand is gotten directly from the sun and reaches the plant easily in an outdoor growing setting. For indoor growers, the grow lights have to be positioned and the plant monitored regularly to ensure that it is getting the adequate amount of light.

Light activates photosynthesis and cannabis grow according to the amount of light that they obtain. They need more light than other plants do, and their growth is dependent on the amount of light that they get among other factors. Parts of the plants where the light does not reach will have stunted growth. Artificial lightning is done by installing huge lamps in the grow area. Grow lights include fluorescent lamps, HID lights and so on. The lights activate the process of photosynthesis for indoor growers and ensure that you get a great yield of buds in the end.

Water

Cannabis need a lot of water to grow. The key to watering cannabis plants is giving them an appropriate amount. Both too little and too much water would hurt the plant. The grower has to water the plants every day without drowning them in it. In the hydroponics method of indoor growing, cannabis is cultivated entirely in water. In outdoor growing also, the plant is constantly searching for water on its own using its roots. All the farmer has to do in such circumstance is simply to sprinkle them with the needed water.

Nutrients

As with cultivating anything, if cannabis do not get the required amount of nutrients, they would not enjoy a robust growth. The proper amount of nutrients that your cannabis needs is often written on the packaging. However, experts recommend that you start with half the amount of nutrients stated. The major nutrients that cannabis need are nitrogen, phosphorus and potassium. They also need calcium, magnesium, iron and copper. Cannabis need more nutrients than most other plants.

For people growing cannabis on their own, they have to ensure that these nutrients are available. For outdoor growing on the other hand, the plant often develops solid roots with which it searches for nutrients on its own. For indoor growers cultivating with soil, it is possible to use a pre-fertilized soil to offer the plant all that it needs. The nutrient requirements of cannabis change with their growing stages. While the plant needs a lot of nitrogen during the vegetative stage, it needs more phosphorus during the flowering stage. A farmer that is effective with his cultivation will ensure that his plants get these nutrients in the right proportion and at the right time.

Temperature

Cannabis plants are sensitive about the temperature of their grow area. They can die from getting frozen and from too much heat thereby bringing the efforts of the grower to nothing. For this to be averted and for the cannabis to grow well, they must be cultivated under room temperature. The temperature could be slightly warmer but not hot or cold. This causes the farmer to regulate how much of light and therefore heat he is giving to the plant. For indoor growers, they can choose to turn off the lights at times of the day when the grow area is really hot. These times could then become the period when the plant requires the lights to be turned off. Cannabis do not need all day lighting. A ratio of sixteen hours of light and eight hours of darkness is usually enough to ensure that the plant is getting enough.

Growing Medium

While the defunct growing method for cannabis and indeed for all plants is soil, it is entirely possible to cultivate without using soil. This is called the soilless method of growing cannabis. For people who are growing cannabis indoors, they often have to choose between using soil or using a soilless method for cultivating their plants. Soilless methods for cultivating cannabis include hydroponics, aeroponics and so on. These basically allow the grower to supply the plant with everything that it needs including nutrients and lighting without dipping them into soil. Notably, soil can also be used for growing cannabis indoors.

The growing method that you choose can affect the container that you use. Once you have determined the method of cannabis cultivation that you prefer, you will need to choose a suitable container for growing it. The appropriate container often depends on the growing method adopted. Growers use anything from small net pots to Rockwool.

Grow Area

This is one of the most important considerations to set into motion before cultivation begins. The grow area could be outdoors or indoors. While growing outdoors, there are no special requirements as to what should be contained in the grow area. The basic thing that the plant needs in an outdoor setting is soil which is already available. Grow areas for indoor cannabis are more varied and largely depend on personal choice. It could be anything from a closet to a part of the basement. The farmer needs to ensure that he will be able to set up the grow area properly. All the essential elements needed for the plant's growth must be able to fit into the grow area. This would include grow lights, grow mediums and so on. When choosing a grow area, the farmer must consider the growing technique that he wants to adopt. When the seeds or clones are ready, he can then begin to set up this grow area to suit the requirements of the plant. Issues such as temperature and how to regulate it will quickly come to play in setting up the grow area.

EFFECTS OF CANNABIS

Cannabis has a lot of accompanying effects. Fortunately, most of these effects are positive. This explains why it is recommended for treatment of different medical ailments. Experts have found that all negative effects of cannabis are simple side effects that do not ignite further medical problems. It is important that we take a look at how cannabis could be good or bad for us.

The Positive Sides of Cannabis

Marijuana may carry different effects for different people. However, there are a couple of common goodness that it brings with it.

➢ Cannabis Causes You To Relax

A lot of people take cannabis because of the soothing effect that it has. Cannabis can make you relax. It does not matter how tensed you are at any point in time. Cannabis can release the tension. If you want something that can calm your nerves at any time, cannabis can do that. It can relax both your body and mind. Medical cannabis is recommended to patients because of its soothing effects. Doctors use cannabis to calm patients down both while treating them and after. This relaxation help that cannabis provides is often activated for disease conditions like epilepsy.

➢ It Ignites Great Sleep

Cannabis is good for getting restful sleep. It ignites a different level of sleep that comes with ease and that its users cannot resist. If you want to sleep like a baby, you can try taking some cannabis. This is why cannabis is recommended for managing insomnia. It goes to work on the nerves and on the brain in a way that relieves you of any pressures and releases comfort hormones that soon transports you to bed.

➢ It Activates Our Creative Juices

Cannabis has been used by creatives to get spectacular work done. Cannabis can drive creativity in a way that creates timeless works of art. If you are finding it difficult to get your creative juices flowing, try taking some cannabis. It would get you started before you know it and you will create some of your best work.

> ➢ **It relieves pain**

Medical cannabis is often recommended for easing pain. It has psychoactive features that help relieve pain. This use for cannabis is so popular that people take their ganja where they want to manage an ongoing pain or do not want to feel pain. For people undergoing chemotherapy, cannabis can be a great way to relieve pain. It does this all while soothing the nerves and giving off a relieving feeling.

> ➢ **It Relieves Nausea**

If you feel nauseous, you might want to take some cannabis. However, this is often recommended based on how severe the nausea is. Cannabis can cause patients to eat by boosting their appetite. This is a very important use for medical cannabis because in many cases, patients may be unable to eat. Doctors can find this easy to deal with using cannabis.

➤ It Reduces Seizures in Epileptic Patients

Easing epilepsy is one of the pivotal uses of cannabis in medicine. Taking marijuana can make epileptic patients feel better. It does this by reducing seizures which then eases the patient. The use of cannabis for epilepsy is popular in children.

➤ It Eases Symptoms of Bipolar Disorder

The effects of cannabis on the brain especially when it gives you a mental high can ease bipolar disorder. Cannabis can stabilize your brain and cause you to relax. In this way, it eases the symptoms of bipolar disorder and is capable of making the patient feel better.

The Negative Sides of Cannabis

Even though the side effects of cannabis are not particularly severe, it is great to know what they are and what to expect with your ganja. Perhaps, there may be some reason why you cannot take it. It is only good that you know. The thing with the side effects of cannabis is that they are almost certain. So, get ready to experience any of these when you take marijuana.

➢ **Increased Appetite**

We have explained above that while helping to cope with nausea, cannabis can also help with the appetite. If you are finding it difficult to eat, marijuana may be the way to go. It leaves you hungry in a way that you have to eat constantly. Before you smoke your buds, make sure to keep some food handy.

➢ **Dry Mouth**

Cannabis inhibits the production of saliva immediately you finish smoking it. This makes the mouth dry. The dryness can be very discomforting but people ease this by chewing on a gum or eating. Don't be surprised when your mouth feels dry after a smoking session. Just keep your solution handy.

➢ **Dizziness**

While sleep is great for you and has already been classified under the positive effects of cannabis, the dizzy feelings that come before it may lend themselves to a different explanation altogether. You could start feeling dizzy before you finish smoking your ganja. This dizziness is said to decrease blood pressure. That would mean that continual dizziness from taking cannabis could lead to problems of its own. For some people, it is easy to resist the dizzy feelings. For others, they would be right in bed within moments. It is important to expect this before you begin smoking cannabis.

Obviously, the side effects of taking cannabis are almost inconsequential beside the positive effects. If you really love your ganja, they should not be enough reasons to deter you. This is even more so when marijuana is to be used as a medical prescription.

Legality of Cannabis

Cannabis is strictly regulated all around the world although we are seeing a relapse in these regulations. The laws governing the use of cannabis are different from one country to another. In certain countries, you can be seen in possession of cannabis and even own it without raising any alarm while in others you cannot. Cannabis is regarded as legal in some countries while it is illegal and outrightly prohibited in others. These differences in legality of cannabis from one place to another can be traced to the prohibitions that occurred in the 1930s and to the changes in those regulations that continue to occur until the present day.

The reasons why the regulations are changing can be traced to the fact that cannabis has continued to prove useful in a lot of important areas.

Medical cannabis falls into this category. It has become necessary to recognize the important role that cannabis plays for curing certain ailments. This has led to more flexible legislations around cannabis. Some laws have stated explicitly that we can use marijuana for medicinal purposes. Good examples are marijuana legislations in Canada, Czech Republic and many other countries. It is quite notable that the legality of marijuana is still an ongoing discussion because medical research continues to follow the pattern of positivity that has been set, and the number of diseases that cannabis is useful for is still an open topic.

There are people who think that since the benefits of marijuana in medicine are serious, there shouldn't be a debate as to its legality. Yet, it is marijuana's rise to relevance that feeds this debate. It becomes important that people check the legality of cannabis in their country or state before owning it. This is a much smaller concern for medical cannabis. If your doctor prescribes it, you will most certainly be within the bounds of the law trying to obtain it. In the next section, we will talk about how marijuana came to assume an important role in man's activities despite it is a plant in the wild.

Cannabis Rise to Popularity

Cannabis is a plant growing in the wild that does not necessarily need human intervention to achieve maximum and robust growth. It has always existed and has had a long interaction with man. It is difficult to say when cannabis came to the attention of humans or how it began growing. In fact, the plant was discovered at different places simultaneously. Discoveries were made when its remains were found in China with traces of the plant in Central Asia also. This has made it impossible to determine when and where marijuana was first found.

One school of thought suggests that cannabis originated in China and then moved from there through human carriers to India and Europe. Another thinks that cannabis can be traced to the TaklaMakan desert which stretches from Caucausus to the Allai massif. Yet another group believes that cannabis was first found between the foothills of the Himalayas and Hindu Kush mountain in South Asia. Researchers in the third group have solid pointers to back their claim as there are several cannabis strains in this region. Also, the people here consume a lot of cannabis. This high consumption and this predominance of cannabis in the area support the claim that cannabis originated there.

Since researchers are not agreed on where cannabis began, we cannot point to a specific place or time. However, we can safely say that cannabis started its journey around the world from Asia. In fact, it is believed that cannabis moved to the rest of the world through immigrants travelling from Asia. As these people moved from one place to another, they taught others how to cultivate, use and enjoy cannabis. Consequently, cannabis became used for a lot of things including meals and textile production. In Medicine, cannabis rose to importance in 2737 BC from the work of Shen Nung who popularized it as one of the parents of medicine in China. Cannabis has been used at different times to alleviate pain. Throughout history, it has found several other uses with the plant going into the manufacturing of fabrics and the construction of the first paper mill in Europe. It then became used for making paper in the next 850 years.

Cannabis followed the Spaniards to Chile and Peru in the 16th century before arriving at Canada and the United States in the 17th century through the British who travelled there. American colonies seized the opportunity to use cannabis for business within the era. The plant then got christened by Carl Linnaeus who called it Cannabis Sativa L. in 1753. After that, a new strain was developed out of the plant by Jean-Baptiste de Lamarck who called it Cannabis Indica. These moves popularized cannabis until 1930 when people began to question how legal the plant was. In 1936, the United States began a silent war against cannabis which culminated in the first cannabis related arrest in 1937. Selling, owning and being in possession of cannabis suddenly became criminal and ignited arrests. In 1942, America removed the use of cannabis from their pharmacology. Cannabis then became banned in several countries. The American President Nixon was at the forefront of the fight against cannabis. He saw the plant as a drug because of its psychoactive features. Following the findings of Dr. Raphael Machoulam in 1964 that listed THC as one of the components of cannabis, President Nixon wanted nothing to do with the plant. This was quickly replicated in other countries that enforced strict rules against cannabis in their territories.

Cannabis was going to see some light in its acceptance following the establishment of a Grow Shop in Holland in 1967 that led to the government decriminalizing it. When Holland took this step, it called for a discourse surrounding the use of cannabis. The legality of cannabis has continued to be called into question all over the world. The lack of a unified agreement on the issue continues to come to play today and is shown in the varying responses by different countries. While cannabis is legal in some places, it isn't in others. In the United States, the legality of cannabis is different from one State to another. Perhaps, the world would reach an agreement on the legality of cannabis as the years go by.

CHAPTER TWO
MEDICINAL CANNABIS

Medicinal cannabis or medicinal marijuana is a therapy that relates to the use of unprocessed cannabis or extracts of it for treating the symptoms of different disease conditions. It is possible to use either a part of the plant or the whole of it in clinical treatment. Medicinal cannabis attests to the fact that marijuana has seen significant progress in its usage in the medical field. It would appear that since being used for medical purposes in early times, the medical value attached to marijuana has only increased. There has been continual breakthrough in the field of medicine as it relates to marijuana.

This medical advancement in relation to marijuana is witnessed side by side its legal battle. Whether that has to do with cultivation, possession or recreational use, cannabis has been long embattled. The medical progress that cannabis has experienced as a plant and which is reminiscent of its use in early times can be applauded. But there is so much ground left to cover.

In the United States, the Food and Drug Administration (FDA) has not given approval or recognition to the use of the marijuana plant in medicine. This is despite scientific advancement in the area. In fact, the FDA has approved two medications containing the chemicals found in marijuana without approving the plant itself or the use of the plant itself. Extracts from cannabis continue to be used for medication which are packaged as pills and which are used for treating different ailments. Cannabis medicine is popular for easing symptoms of disease and the research in this area is still ongoing.

The use of cannabis in medicine is wide ranged. Its chemical components can treat several illnesses and symptoms. It remains rather surprising that something which holds such level of importance is yet to be regarded as legal. A lot of people believe that marijuana should be legal because of its medical significance. As we have seen already, the clamor to make marijuana legal has received attention in a lot of places. Some countries have given the plant and its usage legal backing. The number of states that legalize cannabis in the United States is on the increase. This is replicated around the world and has attracted the attention of medical regulatory bodies worldwide. As it stands, regardless of the upheavals surrounding the legality of cannabis and ethical concerns about its use, the significance of the plant cannot be undermine.

In this chapter, we will go into an exposition of the use of cannabis in medicine to see why it continues to hold a position of relevance.

History of Medicinal Cannabis

Some researchers posit that cannabis has roots reaching as far back as 5,000 years and can be traced to Romania. In spite of the difference of opinion as to where and how cannabis came to us, the collective findings on the subject suggest that cannabis has been around from ancient times. When it comes to its medical usage, there are pointers to the fact that cannabis may have become medically important around 400 AD. Scientists found direct evidence pointing to this possibility from THC found in ashes. The THC is tetrahydrocannabinol and is a component of cannabis. Around 400 AD, people were already using this to ease symptoms of different ailments. Cannabis was used to treat pain and other ailments. When cannabis got to the West, its therapeutic use passed through several transformations including being administered alongside wine. It was also used for the first time to create pills including the drug Marinol which was administered in capsule form. Medicinal cannabis since became popular for being able to alleviate severe pain.

When cannabis got to the United States, it became used as a major pillar of the economy. It was entered in the United States Pharmacopoeia in 1850 and became used as a patent medicine in the 19th and early 20th centuries. Patent medicines were popular for their therapeutic effect throughout the era and medical interest in cannabis was on an upsurge. The use of cannabis in Western medicine was introduced by William Brooke O'Shaughnessy, an Irish Physician. He began using cannabis on animals before moving to his human patients and found that the plant extracts and preparations could ease stomach cramps, muscle spasms and other forms of pain. Doctor Moreau de Tours took this even further with the treatment of migraines and melancholia. He also used the drug as a sleeping aid, an analgesic and an anticonvulsant. The experiments and successful administration of these drugs were not well received outside the medical circle. Strict restrictions were placed on the drugs created using cannabis at a local level so that they were labeled under poison laws where they were to be taken or sold without the prescription of a physician. The regulations that followed immediately were all tilted towards medicinal products and their labeling but they were only a start.

Cannabis was going to be more strictly handled in the mid 19th century despite that there were evidences from its prior history that it could be medically useful. Cannabis became restricted in 1937 when the Marihuana Tax Act was passed. Federal restrictions on use and sale of cannabis were enforced and the plant was subsequently removed from the United States Pharmacopeia in 1942. The legal penalties for possessing cannabis had increased by 1951 with the enactment of the

Boggs Act and further intensified with the enactment of the Narcotic Control Acts of 1956 and the Controlled Substances Act of 1970. While successive American administrations continued to make cannabis criminalized, there was a replication all around the world. These Acts went further to limit cannabis related research by the restriction placed on its procurement. This forestalled the use of cannabis in medicine because medical research was hindered,

The situation turned around at different times around the world with Holland leading the way in 1967. The United States only began to see the need for research into medicinal cannabis in 1996 when California led the way by permitting legal access to botanical cannabis and its usage for medicinal purposes. This access and usage must however be under the supervision of a physician. The State then went ahead to enact the Compassionate Use Act of 1996. This set the pace around the world for the decriminalization of cannabis. Today, cannabis has been approved for recreational use by adults in different countries. It has also been approved for medical use and for cultivation. As we have pointed out, these laws differ from one country to another. The majority of the balance shifts in favor of medicinal cannabis and the potency of cannabis for treating different clinical conditions have long been ascertained.

The facts would however not deter the legal overlords from going after cannabis with even more tempo. Perhaps, it wasn't only the legal concerns that trailed cannabis. As we have seen elsewhere in this book, there were also ethical concerns regarding the use of cannabis medicinally. Experts believed that cannabis had a high abuse potential and there were concerns that people could become dependent on the plant. When these concerns were added to the fact that there were no safety measures for use in place, cannabis continued to remain a somewhat prohibited plant. The only leverage that the plant was allowed because of its enormous significance was medical supervision. In fact, people felt that the use of cannabis only led the way to addiction and misuse of other more harmful substances. Rather than bring medicinal cannabis to an end, these concerns have only allowed for stiffer regulations regarding cannabis use for treatment. Governments and regulatory bodies are continually concerned about how cannabis fits into the framework of drugs and whether it should be included in it at all. From medical certificates to use under prescription, the legal landscape has continued to change for this plant, its extracts and the products made out of it. However, medicinal cannabis has not only thrived but has continued to advance.

CHEMICAL CONSTITUENTS OF CANNABIS

Cannabis became widely used because of its ability to treat several illnesses. Yet, it is not the plant itself or smoking it in the traditional sense that causes these changes. It is the chemicals contained in it that makes this possible. Either by using the plant itself to make medicine or extracting the chemicals in it, scientists and medical researchers have found that cannabis is extremely useful for making drugs that work for different situations. The most common medical use for cannabis is to ease pain. In some cases, this pain can be very severe. Whatever the level of pain experienced by the patient, cannabis and drugs made out of it have been found extremely useful in creating relief. In this section, we would be taking a look at the chemical components of cannabis which make this possible.

What Are Cannabinoids?

Cannabis has a lot of chemical constituents that are unique to it. Although the plant contains a lot of different chemicals, many of these chemicals can also be found in other plants. Medicinal cannabis may have begun with the isolation of active agents in cannabis by 19th century chemists. These chemists were however unable to identify the active component of cannabis. Experts say that this is the case because cannabis lacked nitrogen.

Cannabinoids are chemicals produced from cannabis main component, delta-9-tetrahydrocannabinol (THC). Although THC is cannabis most active component, there are several active components of the plant. Cannabinoids are known to exist only in the cannabis plants. These chemicals are the subject of medical research for controlling certain medical conditions. Some of them are already in use. For example, THC can be used to treat signs and symptoms such as nausea and vomiting and by so doing can relieve a lot of medical conditions associated with these symptoms.

Another important component of cannabis was cannabidiol (CBD) which became the first of its several chemicals to be extracted in its pure form out of the plant. Scientists and illegal manufacturers make cannabinoids in the laboratory and have released many types of cannabinoids making the chemicals up to 100 different types. THC is the ingredient naturally contained in cannabis that creates the body and mental high. THC is a cannabinoid also, and aside the artificially created cannabinoids available, cannabis has its own chemical contents that keep drawing attention to it. Cannabis is a complex plant that has more than 500 chemicals out of which 60 are cannabinoid compounds. It is strikingly interesting that these compounds have opposing effects.

The two major cannabinoids that are relevant to medical practice are THC and CBD. While sativas have high THC content, indicas have high cannabidiol content. A lot of users prefer sativas because of the THC content as it is what gives of the feeling of being high. The preference in medicinal cannabis is based on a different set of ideas entirely as cannabis is used there as a therapy for ailment.

The natural cannabinoid compounds occurring in cannabis are also called phytocannabinoids. THC is the main psychoactive ingredient and the most widely used and distributed of the cannabis compounds. While CBD and THC are similar in certain respects, they are stark opposites in others. Other compounds contained in cannabis include terpenoids, omega fatty acids, flavonoids, and so on. Cannabis gets its aroma from terpenoids as do other flowering plants. Experts have found that some of the effects of cannabis can be traced to terpenoids. While THC can affect a lot of things like emotion, mood, perception, motor function and cognition, CBD are non-psychoactive. Both THC and CBD possess medically useful properties. Wild "feral" cannabis have been found to contain similar amounts of THC and CBD. However, it is more common to find cannabis containing a higher level of THC when compared to its CBD component.

The two most biologically active components of cannabis, THC and CBD also have very different effects on the user. THC can affect the way we think, act or feel. CBD, on the other hand, is the component that has become medically useful because it lessens pain and symptoms such as nausea and vomiting. CBD helps clinical procedures of cancer, multiple sclerosis, neuropathic pain and even pain at the end of life. Thus, CBD helps relieves symptoms associated with chemotherapy in cancer patients, muscle stiffness in spinal cord injury patients as well as low appetite and weight loss in AIDS patients. These uses of the CBD make cannabis itself inevitably important in medicine.

Although cannabis medicine still has a legal battle that it is entangled with, the clinical procedures that CBD helps with have received some legal backing. In many countries and in some states in the United States, cannabis can be used legally to treat Alzheimer's disease, posttraumatic stress disorder, glaucoma, chronic pain, cancer, severe nausea, Crohn's disease, epilepsy, multiple sclerosis, ALS, hepatitis C, seizures, chronic weight loss. Even though cannabis can be use legally to treat these conditions, scientists have not found evidences that point to cure using cannabis for all of these conditions. Research is still underway to determine which of these conditions cannabis actually helps. It is however clear that cannabis is effective as a painkiller. This makes it effective for use during chemotherapy and other similar conditions that we have mentioned elsewhere in this book. The fact that cannabis can act as and is being used as a superior drug for certain conditions is simply phenomenal. It is indeed the focus of medical cannabis. Hopefully, the number of conditions that cannabis can treat will increase with time, and with the relaxing of governmental regulations around cannabis in a way that makes production and research possible.

Cannabis has a lot of different strains as we have discussed in the preceding chapter. All these strains have both THC and CBD content. It is the responsibility of the grower that he takes care of the plant during the growing process in a way that leads to a buoyant yield of THC and CBD. All the other chemicals contained in cannabis work together to make it a great plant for use in medicine. In fact, one research showed that CBD was more effective when mixed with other biological non-cannabinoid components of cannabis than when it was used in its pure form. The different cannabis strains have different THC to CBD ratio and the component that is higher determines how that strain would react when used. If there is more THC in it, you are more likely to get the mind-altering high feeling that is capable of affecting your judgment, mood and memory. If the CBD content is higher, the strain becomes even more greater in its medical effects. Depending on what health problem cannabis is to be used for, each cannabis component can be very useful. Your health care provider is in the proper position to recommend which medicinal cannabis suits your condition.

Although the unique chemical components of cannabis are at least 60, these components do not necessarily have different effects. Most of them are closely related and they have been grouped into 10 according to their interactions. Experts say that a lot of these chemical constituents differ by only a single chemical moiety and may share biochemical pathways even in their byproducts.

Differing Characteristics of Cannabis' Chemical Constituents

It was the psychoactive effects of cannabis that made it popular because the plant was mind-altering in a pleasurable way. However, it has numerous chemical constituents that are not psychoactive. In fact, of the over 400 chemicals that have been identified in the plant, more than 300 have nothing to do with making you feel high. How do we differentiate these chemical components and their effects? We will discuss the more important ones in this section.

THC and CBD are the most researched of the cannabis components. They have been widely researched in both animals and humans and there are solid pointers to their effects. According to experts, THC produces hypoactivity, hypothermia, spatial and verbal short term memory impairment in a dose dependent manner. CBD, on the other hand, does not have such effects on the human body. Thus, it is non-psychoactive. While THC affects memory, locomotor activity, and temperature, CBD does not have the same effect. In fact, higher doses of CBD can lower the effects of THC where the later is much lower. Researchers agree that although CBD and THC may be the same in many respects, they are also different in so many others. These differences have been scientifically proven in a lot of instances. In an early study, both compounds were administered to 40 healthy volunteers while researchers measured their pulse rate and psychological reactions. In the results that followed, THC increased pulse rate and induced strong psychological reactions while CBD did not. Instead of producing adverse effects of its own, CBD blocked many of the effects of THC. The combination of both compounds produced pleasurable feelings in the subjects.

These studies have continued today to dig into individual and collective effects of THC and CBD. Researchers are carrying out double-blind pseudo-randomized studies on healthy volunteers who had previously been exposed to cannabis. Participants were administered THC and CBD along with placebo (flour) and given verbal memory tasks, emotional tasks, inhibition tasks and auditory and visual sensory processing tasks. The results obtained showed that both compounds had differing effects on all levels and even exhibited opposing brain activation in some parts of the brain. While THC increased anxiety levels, intoxication and sedation, CBD had no such effects. THC also caused momentary psychotic symptoms that CBD did not. There were no serious changes to behavior ignited by CBD.

In another study, the findings showed that CBD could prevent the transient psychotic symptoms induced by THC where it was used prior to introducing THC. It would appear therefore that both components continue to balance each other. A recent study shows that CBD could significantly reduce anxiety and treat social anxiety disorder by acting on limbic and paralimbic areas of the brain. The culmination of these studies has led to the proposition that CBD has antipsychotic effects and may be a potential antipsychotic medicine. Medical experts are currently developing the compound into a medicine for several conditions including diabetes, cancer, inflammation and neurodegenerative diseases.

It is important to know that these anti-THC effects that CBD has are not peculiar to it. The same interaction between cannabis constituents can also be observed with the compound tetrahydrocannabivarin (d-9-THCV). This compound is potentially useful for treating obesity and epilepsy. Studies show that THCV produces anti-obesity effects by working against the appetite surge that comes with cannabis consumption. Instead of the compound to help patients take less food, it increases their energy expenditure in a way that causes them to lose weight. A notable researcher on the subject has even gone further to show that d-9-THCV has the potential to manage other disorders such as chronic liver disease where these disorders are associated with inflammation.

The chemical constituents of cannabis work together to provide the high feeling that is striking about the plant while balancing the effects that this has on the brain. More importantly, they help to make medicinal cannabis possible. The compounds which do these are the cannabinoids which are the peculiar 60 compounds found in cannabis alone. Indeed, researchers are still looking out for more ways in which cannabinoids can be used for medical treatment. Recent studies in animals show that marijuana extracts can be used to kill some cancer cells and reduce others. When such extracts were administered to rodents in a cell culture study, researchers found that growth of cancer cells was slowed. The cancer cells targeted in this study were related to brain tumors. Another research in mice showed that purified extracts of THC and CBD increased the potency of radiation for killing cancer cells.

Both preclinical and clinical trials are underway using marijuana and extracts from it to treat symptoms of various disease conditions. Some of the conditions that marijuana has proven for include multiple sclerosis, HIV/AIDS, seizures, inflammation, pain, substance abuse disorders, mental disorders, and so on. Cannabinoid medications are used to treat nausea resulting from chemotherapy. As we have pointed out above, CBD can be used to treat obesity. Similarly, current cannabinoid medications are being used to increase appetite for weight loss patients in extreme conditions. In the United States, the Food and Drug Administration (FDA) have approved the drugs, dronabinol and nabilone, both of which contain THC to treat nausea caused by chemotherapy and to induce appetite for extreme weight loss caused by AIDS. The medication nabiximols (Sativex®) has also been approved in several European countries including the United Kingdom and Canada to treat muscle control problems. This medication is a mouth spray that contains THC and CBD.

The two major components of cannabis may differ in their effects but have been consistently used in medicinal cannabis to ease several symptoms and make ailments better.

Risks Associated with Medical Cannabis

The chemicals contained in cannabis work in our bodies by connecting with specific parts of our cells that are called receptors. For the chemicals to work and their effects to manifest, they have to reach what scientists call your cannabinoid receptors. These receptors are situated in cells residing in your brain and in your immune system. The process of how cannabinoids affect the cannabinoid receptors is still unclear. However, all the medical effects of cannabis and even its detrimental effects are activated by first reaching our cannabinoid receptors. Both THC and CBD have to connect with specific receptors in our brain and immune system for their effects to manifest.

Although cannabis is great for easing nausea, pain and other symptoms, frequent use can lead to other problems. Similarly, cannabis cannot be used alongside all other medicines. It may not interact well with those medicines. These include medicines that control your mood and induce sleep. Hence, you cannot use cannabis with sedatives, antidepressants, anxiety medication and opioids. Cannabis can also not be used with alcohol and tobacco. The effect of the medicine would usually determine whether or not you can use cannabis along with it. Once you have determined that a particular medicine might be altering in one form or the other, you can skip taking it along with your cannabis medicine. Cannabis can work well with so many other medicines. This is why medical prescription is important before taking cannabis. Your doctor would be able to tell you which medicines can be combined with cannabis and which ones cannot be.

If you take medicine for blood pressure, you may want to skip cannabis medicines. Cannabis can alter your blood pressure and make the situation worse. For people on blood thinners, cannabis increases the chances of bleeding. It becomes important that your doctor knows all the other medications you use before recommending cannabis to you. Tell your doctor about all the other medicines that you take. If there is a substance abuse history in your family, your health care provider should know that also. If there are mental health disorders as well, you should let your doctor know. The THC content of cannabis can make these situations worse. Cannabis is capable of affecting your memory, concentration, judgment, coordination and decision making. You may put yourself at risk if you drive after using cannabis. This is the same with operating machinery of other kind. If you are on cannabis medication, you can handle machinery in a harmful manner. Since the components of cannabis balance out each other and have different effects, your health care provider is the appropriate person to tell you if cannabis use is proper in a particular situation. Ask your doctor or other health care provider if it is safe for you to drive while using cannabis. As we have seen in the previous chapters, there are specific side effects to expect from cannabis use. These include dry mouth, dizziness, drowsiness, nausea and vomiting. Other side effects include faster heart rate, red eyes, anxiety or paranoid thoughts. The effects of cannabis experienced may differ from one person to another.

A major risk associated with cannabis use is nausea and vomiting. This is called cannabinoid hyperemesis syndrome, or CHS. It is ignited when cannabis is used long term and on a regular basis. The condition causes thirst, diarrhea and stomach cramps. It comes with bouts of vomiting that lasts over 24 hours and continues throughout the day. Medical cannabis should be used in pregnancy and during breastfeeding only after speaking to a health care practitioner on the safety of doing so. Cannabis use during pregnancy and breastfeeding may affect the proper development and the health of your baby.

A condition known as cannabis use disorder may arise may follow regular use. It could range from mild to severe. People who have cannabis use disorder continue to take cannabis despite any harmful effects they may be experiencing. Cannabis use disorder could follow where it is used every day, the user has other substance use disorders or mental health disorders, or where he had begun using it at a young age.

Researchers have found that cannabis use can lead to psychotic disorders such as schizsophrenia.

Similarly, stopping cannabis use can lead to withdrawal symptoms. The user may develop sleep troubles, anxiety and intense craving to use cannabis. In some form of medicinal cannabis, some of these risks may be absent because cannabis is diluted into oils, creams or pills. The associated risks may be much higher where cannabis is taken in its raw forms. If you smoke medical cannabis, there are the more serious risks of developing chronic cough or bronchitis which can damage your lungs.

There are also ways to reduce the risk that comes with using cannabis. Even though these risks are not automatic, it is great to take some precautions. If you want to lower your risks for developing any of the conditions discussed, you should consider speaking with your health care provider before you use cannabis. Make sure that you have a complete history of your drug use on hand so that you do not leave anything out as some drugs cannot be combined with cannabis. Avoid taking cannabis along with alcohol and tobacco. Avoid driving and do not operate any machinery while you are on medical cannabis as this can lead to your involvement in a car crash. Research has successfully linked cannabis use to car accidents, so this is something you would not want to try.

Although cannabis can interact well with a lot of medicines, it is safer to reduce this interaction. Do not use cannabis with any medicines that will only aggravate its effects such as medicines meant to control sleep, blood pressure and mood. You can talk to your health care provider about using cannabis medicines that have lower THC content. If there is more CBD to THC ratio in the product, you will automatically reduce many of the risks associated with cannabis use. You should store your cannabis medicines properly. For edible cannabis, you want to keep them away from children to avoid the risk of them equating the medicines with snacks. Keep them in a secure place where only you can access. If a problem arises in the course of using cannabis medicine, you should contact your health care provider immediately.

CHAPTER THREE

CANNABIS MEDICINES

We have said a lot about the fact that cannabis has become an effective medical ingredient for drugs easing pain and other symptoms. We have also looked at the historical perspective of how cannabis got there. We are yet to discuss the specific ways cannabis is used medically. Does the user have to swallow a pill? If he does, is medicinal cannabis always available in pill form?

The effects of cannabis begin to manifest depending on the method by which it is taken. This also determines how long the effects last. Cannabis can be smoked, brewed as tea, inhaled, sprayed under the tongue, applied to the skin or eaten in homemade food. When cannabis is smoked, the effects manifest within minutes. When it is eaten, its effects may take up to ninety minutes to begin to manifest. As a result, medical cannabis would naturally come with instructions on how to use. Are all these methods applicable to medical cannabis? When we refer to medicinal cannabis, what in precise terms are we talking about?

In this chapter, we would be taking a look at the various cannabis medicines that are available in the field.

Different Kinds of Cannabis Medicines

While the dried flower or bud from a mature female cannabis plant can be used to create medicines, the more popular form of cannabis medicines around the world are gotten from extracts or concentrates of the cannabis plant. These concentrates are derived from cannabinoid-rich glandular trichomes. These trichomes are found on the flowers, leaves and stalks of the cannabis plant. The greater amount of trichomes can be found on the flowers of a mature female cannabis plant. There are a lot of methods used to extract the trchomes from the plant but that's not the subject of this discourse.

Cannabinoids are capable of dissolving when placed in fats, alcohol, oils, water and butters. Thus, they are said to be fat-solluble hydroponic oils. Using any of these agents, cannabinoids can be extracted from the cannabis plant. Let's take a look at the various preparations that are cannabis medicines and how they can be used.

Cannabis Edibles

Cannabis can be added to food. It can be brewed and taken as tea or other beverage. It can be eaten along with cake, cookies, and dressings.

Cannabis is made edible by heating its extracts or concentrates during which process the THC is converted from its acid form into active THC. Various forms of converted cannabis can be used to make edible cannabis medications. The amount of cannabinoid used in making the edible cannabis determines its potency.

Cannabis Butter

Cannabis butter is also called cannabutter. It is butter infused with cannabinoids. To get cannabutter, raw cannabis is heated to extract cannabinoids into the butter. This can be achieved by heating the cannabis and butter mixture over low temperature. You can use a frying pan, a pot or a slow cooker to achieve this. Cannabutter can be taken as edible cannabis by adding it to any recipe that includes oil and does not go over 280 degrees Fahrenheit.

Cannabis Oil

Cannabis oil, also called cannaoil, is cooking oil infused with cannabinoids. The cannabinoids is extracted by heating the oil and cannabis together over low temperature. This can be done using a frying pan, a pot, a double boiler or a slow cooker. Following the same process as with the cannabutter, you then strain out the plant material from the mixture. This can be used in any recipe that includes oil and does not go beyond 280 degrees Fahrenheit. You can use this oil with candies, cakes and food of all kinds.

Hash Oil

Hash oil is made from essential oils and resins (trichomes) extracted from the leaves of a mature cannabis plant. The oils and resins are extracted using various solvents like ethanol and hexane which are subsequently evaporated. Hash oil has a lot of cannabinoids and its THC content can range from thirty to ninety percent. The oil can be taken through a pipe, a vaporizer or added to food.

Hashish

This is also known as hash or hashish. It is made with a collection of concentrated or compressed trichomes. Interestingly, hash is more potent than the cannabis plant itself. It has the same volume of cannabinoids as the foliage from which it is made but in even higher concentrations. Hashish is different in hardness from one to the other. It is a paste-like substance that is pliable and soft. It only gets hardened as it oxidizes and the oil evaporates. It also gets less potent in the process. Hashish contains a THC content of fifteen to seventy percent. It can be smoked with a pipe, can be eaten along with food, used with a vaporizer or mixed with aromatic herbs.

Kief

This is a powder-like substance that is made from trichomes. The trichomes are gotten from the flowers and leaves of the cannabis plant. Klef can be used to make cakes or can be consumed as a powder smoked through a pipe. Kief can also be consumed along with cannabis buds and other herbs.

Cannabis Topicals

This is a mixture created by combining cannabinoids with a penetrating topical cream. The cream is then applied to the skin reaching directly into the affected areas of the body and penetrating deep into body tissues. Cannabis tropicals can be applied to areas of the skin with allergic reactions. It can also be applied to any muscle strain, inflammation or swelling. Topical cannabis cream can relieve pain and reduce inflammation. The THC and CBD content work together to make this happen. This kind of cannabis medicine is not psychoactive unlike the effects that you get through inhaling or eating.

Cannabis topical includes salves and creams. Salves are heated into coconut oil combined with bees wax and then cooled afterwards. They can be rubbed directly on the skin. Cannabis topical creams are created by heating cannabinoids into shea butter. This can also be applied directly on the skin once cooled. This cannabis medicine has been used for psoriasis, some types of dermatitis, fever blisters, herpes, lip balms, acne, pains caused by rheumatism and arthritis, hemorrhoids, migraines, and so on.

Pharmaceutical Cannabis

These are pharmaceutical pills with standardized doses, composition and formulation. You can easily measure the amount of cannabinoid you are getting with each dose. Pharmaceutical cannabis can also come in sprays. These are also regulated and adhere to all the requirements prescribed by physicians.

Cannabis Liquor

You can infuse liquor with cannabinoids just as you did with butter and cooking oil. This can be added to coffee and other beverages. The best way to consume it is to cook stems and leaves of cannabis into brandy or rum.

Tincture

This is made by using ethanol alcohol such as pure grain alcohol to extract the cannabinoids. This is then absorbed through the mucous membranes in droplet amounts.

Spray

This is an extension of tinctures. After extracting the cannabinoids through ethanol alcohol, the solution derived is then sprayed under the tongue using a spray. Sublingual sprays have pumps that make this really easy to achieve.

Sativex®

This has been approved for alleviating all kinds of symptoms including neuropathic pain, overactive bladder, spasticity and symptoms of cancer. This comes in form of a mouth spray and its legality as with all things cannabis depends on the country. This medication was made from two strains of cannabis. The active components include THC and CBD and they are used to make this oromucosal spray when they are suspended in ethanol. The prescription contains a dose of 2.7mg THC and 2.5mg CBD with each spray.

Dronabinol (Marinol®)

Dronabinol (Marinol®) is another medication that has been popularly prescribed. It comes in a capsule and has been classified in the United States as a Schedule III drug. It is used to treat nausea and vomiting that results from chemotherapy in cancer patients, and loss of weight and appetite in AIDS patients. This medication is made by suspending THC in sesame oil. It does not contain CBD or any other cannabinoid.

How to Use Cannabis Medicines

From the foregoing, it is obvious that the various cannabis medicines offer different methods of usage. Although the cannabinoids interact with CB1 and CB2 receptors all over the body, the method for taking them isn't that uniform. The method by which you take each cannabis medicine can also affect the intensity of the effects that you feel just as much as the volume of the cannabinoids used does. Each of these methods is an effective method to use cannabis but of course you cannot inhale the creams. You have to apply that. The form in which medical cannabis comes can therefore determine how it is applied.

Ingesting

Cannabis can be ingested by eating the medicine. In fact, this is the safest way to take the medication. When you ingest cannabis, it may take an hour or more for the effects to manifest and they last longer than if you had inhaled them. Eating them also allows cannabinoids to go through the digestive process. This metabolizes the chemical components differently than if you had inhaled them. The effects are also said to be different and are subjective to the individual. It would take experimentation with different product types and dosages to eventually find the appropriate edible cannabis medication that is effective for each individual. It is advisable that you increase the dose little by little while starting with small amounts that you allow two hours to be properly ingested. You can ingest cannabis pills and put in the effort to find the appropriate dosage for you.

Direct Application

As we have seen, cannabis topicals are better used by direct application on the affected areas of the skin. In fact, this cannot be applied any other way. This is a safe method for consuming cannabis. It may be preferred for some people and is even the best option for certain ailments especially where pain is the major target of the medication.

Cannabis applied directly on the skin does not activate any psychoactive effects.

Inhaling

Cannabis medicine can also be consumed by inhalation. There are certain forms of cannabis medicines that cannot be used without inhalation. However, you can choose how you want to inhale the medicine. There are different methods of inhalation. We will discuss these methods in this section of the book.

Inhale by Smoking

Smoking the medication works really fast when compared to other methods. As a result, the effects can be felt quickly and relief happens fast. The problem with going the smoking route is that you may be at least of coughing severely because of potential irritants inhaled alongside from the tars. It is advisable that you smoke cannabis as little as possible if you intend to inhale it through this method. It is advisable that you smoke cannabis as little as possible per time. Experts suggest that you try 1 to 3 inhalations at a time and wait for 10 to 15 minutes to find the dosage that works for you.

Inhaling through a Pipe

You can inhale cannabis through a pipe. You can choose between different pipes. However, if you are using a water pipe, it is important that you don't do that regularly. The reason for this is that you can inhale water vapor or drops in the process. You should go for glass pipes, brass pipes or stainless steel pipes. If you are inhaling with a bong, you should avoid those made from rubber, plastic or aluminium. These can produce harmful fumes if they get melted or heated in the process. You should change the water frequently to avoid inhaling germs and other impurities.

Inhale through a Vaporizer

A vaporizer will heat the oils and transform them into airborne vapors all while keeping the rest of the plant material. In this way, the vaporizer reduces the amount of tars and other chemical irritants that you would have inhaled. This reduces the risks for harsh coughing and other lung problems. Vaporizers emit fewer odors than smoking cannabis any other way. A hand-held vaporizer is great for inhaling cannabis. You can even make your own vaporizer if you are unable to buy one.

Alternative Treatments in Cannabis Medicine

Aromatherapy and Homeopathy are alternative medical treatments. They have become popular from being used in addition to conventional Western Medicine. Like other alternative medicines, these two focus on the underlying cause of pain and illness. Instead of merely making an illness better, alternative medicine focuses on the root cause and deals with this once and for all. Aromatherapy and Homeopathy are alternative medicines that are related to cannabis medicine. They are treatments designed to boost the immune system and speed healing. We cannot discuss cannabis medicine in full without venturing into these two.

Aromatherapy

Aromatherapy is a treatment that focuses on using essential oils extracted from the bark, flowers, leaves and roots of the cannabis plant to provide relief. It is healing initiated by the therapeutic use of pure essential oils. The treatment regimen targets health and balance and works to heal the body, mind, skin and emotions. Aromatherapy offers both psychological and physiological benefits to our health. Aromatherapy works with several plants and is not restricted to cannabis alone. The parts of a plant can be used for various treatment methods that are focused on healing and on overall health. Some of the ways that aromatherapy has been used include diffusing eucalyptus oil to help ease congestion. The essential oils are extracted from the plant through steam distillation.

The oils made during aromatherapy called essential oils can be inhaled or applied on the skin. They help to relieve pain and can increase cognitive function. They also act well as mood enhancers. Essential oils are not properly regulated for medical treatments. As a result, it is important that you put in the research to find out what you are buying. In cannabis medicine, aromatherapy can be used to make essential oils and cannabis topical that are then applied directly to the skin to enhance healing. These are used by applying them directly to the part of the body where the patient is experiencing pain. Cannabis is known for its pain relieving effects that are almost instantaneous. Through aromatherapy, patients with clinical conditions such as pain receive respite faster than conventional Western medicine pills.

Homeopathy

Homeopathy is a principle that states that introducing small doses of a substance to the body can induce healing. The medication introduced can stimulate the body to heal itself. Homeopathy also stipulates that medication is more effective with lower doses. Homeopathy is based on the principle that says "like cures like" and it administers minute doses of natural substances based on the individuality of the patient and the peculiarity of the illness such as its severity. Homeopathy is regarded as both an art and a science and was first developed by German doctor Samuel Hahnemann in 1810. Although homeopathy was used extensively in Europe and America for more than 200 years, it experienced a decline in the USA as a result of the emergence of modern medicine. Homeopathy has now begun to regain its popularity across the USA. Homeopathy is accepted all over the world as a safe alternative to modern medicine.

It is a natural supplement for optimizing general health and well being. The minute doses from the plants are used to stimulate the immune system. Treatments designed with homeopathy are customized to suit the needs of each individual. Homeopathy remedies come as gels, tablets, pellets, creams, drops, and ointments. The remedies are consumed by inhaling, ingesting or placing the pellets under your tongue. Homeopathic remedies can cure conditions such as bruises, skin irritations, hormonal imbalance, muscle cramps, back pain, gastrointestinal problems and so on. It can also cure psychological and behavioral problems like phobias and addictions.

CHAPTER FOUR

CLINICAL USES OF CANNABIS

Cannabis can be used to treat a number of severe clinical conditions. As we pointed out in Chapter two of this book, it does this by connecting with the cannabinoid receptors in our brains. We have the CB1 and CB2 receptors among others all over our bodies even in our skin. In this chapter, we will consider specific clinical conditions and how they interact with cannabis.

CLINICAL CONDITIONS AND THEIR INTERACTION WITH CANNABIS

While cannabis can be used to treat medical symptoms, there are clinical conditions that it can be used to ameliorate. These conditions include depression, stress, anxiety, sleep disorders and chronic pain. We have already emphasized the use of cannabis to ease pain throughout this book. Medicinal cannabis goes beyond just relieving symptoms in many cases to actually treating the conditions. In this section, we will talk discuss the clinical conditions and move on to how cannabis interacts with them to make the situation better.

DEPRESSION

There is a thin line between being depressed and being sad. The intensity at which this sadness occurs and the fact that it happens for prolonged periods are some of the things that point us towards depression. We know that this may be more than sadness because it never goes away. No matter what we do, we cannot motivate ourselves. Depression goes beyond feeling unhappy and unmotivated for a few days. It is persistent and can last up to several weeks or months at a time. Depression can seize the joy out of your life. It can make you despair yourself. It is debilitating and takes charge of your day. When you are living with depression, it can feel like you are just passing the time. You can feel like nothing is going right in your life. The downside is that while you are letting yourself go due to depression, you become unable to utilize your time correctly. You stay distracted, and everything that once gave you joy now feels like a burden. The sadness that comes with depression is deep. Your thinking is affected, and your general well being will be in jeopardy. When you are depressed, you achieve your goals more slowly. You spend a lot of time wallowing in feelings of hopelessness, and you achieve less in a lot of time. Depression is a time killer, but this is not its most memorable trait. It impairs your mental health and makes you see yourself and your life as worthless.

One in ten people struggles with depression throughout their lives. The statistics make depression a severe health problem. It cuts across genders and ages, and anyone could become prone to depression. It has been indicated that around four percent of children between ages five and sixteen in the UK are depressed. The mental health condition continues to impact people all over the world.

Depression can fizzle out and arise again throughout a person's life. It can get a lot worse with each episode, and it can get better. It can begin to ease right after a terrible episode. As a result, it is essential that you start treating depression as soon as you discover its first signs. Treatment for depression doesn't end on one encounter. It is a continuous process. You must continue to get support, and you must continue to take what is called maintenance treatment to ensure that your symptoms don't return. If you do not want a relapse, you would want to get the right support and treatment. Some experts believe that despite assertions that depression cannot be cured, it is possible to recover fully from the illness. There are serious medical links between cure and cannabis. However, cannabis is not the only way to go about treating depression. In fact, in many cases, it may not be part of the doctor's prescription. We will explain the other methods for treating depression in the pages that follow. One of such treatment methods and a vital one is medication.

According to The American Psychiatric Association, it is best to continue to take your current medication for between four to nine months once your first depressive episode is alleviated. This will reduce your risk of a reoccurrence. It is difficult to determine whether you have depression because there are no particular set of signs pointing towards depression. The condition manifests differently for everyone. Some people exhibit anxiety, while others do not. The broad symptoms include feelings of hopelessness, sadness, disinterest and anxiety. You can even become stressed out as a result of depression. You can feel stressed without any actual evidence to warrant this state. If you have perpetual moments of feeling down, it may be time for you to figure out whether you have depression. Being sure about this is the first step to overcoming the mental health condition and to actual self-care.

In the next section, we will go into an exposition of the signs and symptoms of depression. Depression is not one of those things you should allow in your life. It is something that needs to be nipped in the bud. The moment you suspect that you have depression, you should begin to seek cure. If your symptoms are adequately managed, you should be able to overcome depression. If you are feeling down or going through perpetual moments of sadness, you would want to decide whether what you are going through is depression or just momentary sadness.

Depression Triggers

Medical practitioners have found that there may be several causes for depression instead of a single cause. Several factors could work together to trigger depression. These triggers depend on the person involved, including their gender, age, sex, and so on. The causes of depression can be unrelated. They can also include a series of traumatic or stressful life events. Money worries and ailment can cause depression. The stress that you feel from a significant illness can trigger depression even after you have recovered. If you are always worrying about money, you can become depressed. The situation is the same as other life situations like a divorce. The causes of depression, therefore, really depend on what is going on in our lives.

Some of the factors that can play in a role in igniting depression include psychological and social factors, environmental factors, genetic factors, changes in the brain's neurotransmitter levels, and so on. Doctors and the rest of the medical community are yet to understand why people get depressed. While some people think that depression is a trivial issue, evidence continues to show that depression is a serious condition and that it affects a lot of people. Common depression triggers include loneliness, a family history of depression, illness and recovery, stressful events as we have pointed out, childbirth, grief, and so on. Anything capable of making you feel a dramatic and sudden change in the progression of your life can cause depression. Depression is your response to the new situation and a way that you react to all that is going on around you. The fact that this response may be unfavorable usually comes under the list.

People who have a family history of depression or another mood disorder have a higher risk of depression. Childhood trauma can also cause depression later in life because such events work to determine how a person's body responds to stress and fearful situations. Scientists have also linked brain inactivity that results from the brain structure to depression. There is no confirmed stance as to whether the inactivity of the frontal lobe of the brain that is witnessed during depression is a cause of depression or a result of its symptoms. In the same manner that depression can cause complications where certain medical conditions are present, it may result from other medical conditions too. If you have attention-deficit hyperactivity, insomnia, chronic pain or illness, you may be at risk for depression. Inappropriate use of drugs and alcohol can also lead to depression. The evidence in this regard shows that about twenty-one per cent of people who have a history of substance abuse go through depression. If you are in this bracket, you may become depressed soon. Low self-esteem and self-criticism are other factors that can lead to depression. People with a history of other mental illness may become depressed. Depression can also be a side effect of certain medications as we have pointed out elsewhere in this book. It is entirely possible for a person to interact with any of these triggers and not develop depression. Also, the cause of depression is different from one person to another. There are a lot of situations in which the cause of depression was not deciphered. In many ways, depression takes a personal stance. You should stay away from the triggers that have been identified where you can.

Identifying Your Triggers

Depression is different for everyone. It manifests in different ways for people going through it. The symptoms of depression can be starkly opposite. While one person may have insomnia, another can be sleeping way too much. Its triggers are varied between people also. It is essential that you know what your depression triggers are to be able to get the help you need. That could be difficult if you have never been depressed before. If you have had one depressive episode in the past, you should be able to identify what led to that and avoid a reoccurrence. If your depression resulted from worries over money, you could start taking more control of your money so that you don't go down that hole again.

Similarly, you should take note of your symptoms. This would make the process more manageable when you are consulting with a doctor. Are you feeling increasingly fatigued? Are you experiencing sharp deviations with your weight and appetite? Are you restless and agitated? Is your speech slowed? Have you lost interest in the things that once gave you joy? Are you more irritable than is healthy for you? Do you have trouble concentrating? Is your decision making disturbed? Is your sleep routine distorted? Do you feel guilty, hopeless, helpless or anxious? Do you feel empty like there is something missing within you? Do you have digestive issues and suffer from physical aches and pain? Do you often think of dying? Take note of all these conditions before your appointment with a doctor as they are indicative of depression. Do not assume that they will go away with time. Where you have given them time, and they are persistent, you have a problem on your hands that you need to deal with immediately. Do not hesitate to seek help with your situation.

Before your doctor would diagnose these symptoms like depression, they must be occurring for most of your day. Are you going through any of these for up to two weeks and every day within those two weeks? Stop assuming. You need to see a doctor already. You do not need to manifest all the symptoms before you can be depressed. You do not even need to have most of the symptoms. A few of the symptoms are enough to show that the condition exists. If you discover that you are having any of the symptoms, you should see a healthcare professional immediately. If you are having a second depressive episode, the symptoms may be simpler than the first time you experienced the illness. They would also be easy to recognize. They could be as simple as sleeping for longer than usual.

It is normal to worry about a reoccurrence if you have gone through depression before. If you find yourself thinking about your risk of getting depressed all over again, you should see your doctor and your therapist immediately. They will let you know what you should watch out for, and they will make it easy to prevent depression from happening all over again. Your treatment team already knows what your risk factors are and can be very helpful in avoiding a second depressive episode. We will go through a quick exposition on depression in this section of the book before exploring how cannabis can help. We will also take you the interactions between different medical conditions. Conditions like anxiety, depression and insomnia can get interwoven. They can even result in further complications that are in fact other more serious medical conditions. By going through this exposition, you will understand how each of these conditions can lead to the other and how cannabis can help. Depending on what condition you are treating however, it is often a great idea for you to talk to your doctor to determine whether you can use cannabis, what dose of cannabis is good for you and in what proportions.

SHOULD YOU MANAGE YOUR DEPRESSION SYMPTOMS OR SEEK CURE?

Now that you know what your symptoms are, what would be the appropriate action to take? It is possible to manage your symptoms such as by removing the cause of the sadness. Also, we have pointed out that depression does not have a cure. What treatment can do for you is remission. In some cases, depression eventually leaves. In other cases, it lingers, or it reoccurs. When you consider this, you may be hesitant about approaching a physician to treat your symptoms.

Some people also experience uncontrollable feelings of shame. You may feel that your depressive moods are just so terrible and may not want to discuss them with somebody else. You may want to keep your sad feelings and your symptoms to yourself. Depression is not something to be ashamed of or to hide. It is something to work through and to tackle as soon as you discover that it may be present. The earlier you get your symptoms diagnosed, the earlier you will get as much help as you need.

Do not try to manage your depression symptoms on your own. Check in with a medical practitioner or a mental health professional. Your doctor or therapist will help you confirm the state of your symptoms as well as whether what you are experiencing is depression at all. Reading books like this is a first step to overcoming depression. You need all the information you can access to tackle this and to make your symptoms subside. You should not let yourself suffer when it has been confirmed that depression is a highly treatable illness. Treatment has worked for a lot of people. Who is to say it would not work for you? Avoid self-management of depression and give yourself the very best by booking that appointment right now!

Some health conditions can get worse as a result of depression. If you have any of these conditions and do not seek treatment for your depression, you can expose yourself to further complications. Such medical conditions include asthma, cancer, arthritis, diabetes, cardiovascular disease and obesity. These medical conditions can develop into more significant health problems if you neglect depression treatment. Feeling down can be a reaction to upsetting events and is a normal part of life. However, if you are regularly sad to the extent that it has become your default state, you should consider checking with a doctor. Your primary care doctor will confirm if you are indeed normal or are suffering from depression. If you do not get adequate treatment, depression itself will get worse. With the right treatment, however, you can begin to see improvements. Your symptoms will ease, and you will feel better. The best part is that you will feel the result of treatment in just a few weeks.

SIGNS OF DEPRESSION

Depression can be averted if you discover it early. This is why it is essential to know what its symptoms are. Depression is more than being in the blues. It is more than being always sad. When we are sad, we can quickly engage in activities that lighten us up. This is not the case for a person who is depressed. They are usually unable to partake in such activity, and when they do, they are likely to find no joy in it. A general lack of energy characterizes depression. It can come with a lot of symptoms that are more than just sadness, and that is simultaneous. A person who is depressed can manifest a lot of different signs at the same time. The symptoms of depression can vary based on age and gender. Also, they often manifest unconsciously. What a woman may experience when she is depressed can be different from what a man would experience. The same goes for children as well. This makes it difficult to pin the symptoms of depression to specifics. In spite of these, there are some signs of depression that are common to everyone going through the condition. Some of the symptoms of depression are common to everyone whether or not we are going through depression. With depressed individuals, the symptoms are more intensified and are multiplied. They occur over more extended periods, are strongly expressed, and numerous symptoms can be combined. When a person is excessively anxious, for example, we can say that they are depressed. If anxiety is an isolated event that quickly subsides, however, depression would not be the right tag to give the situation. It can be instead an incident of feeling low that quickly passes, and this is normal with everyone.

If the symptoms of depression do not persist, then what you are going through is just temporary feelings of low energy. You could just be having a bad mood. We all go through such emotions when we are going through difficult times in our lives. This mood quickly changes, too and there is usually a quick improvement in the way that we feel and the way we approach our daily life. For depression, the reverse is the case, and bad moods only get worse.

You could experience tiredness all the time along with a lack of sex drive, loss of appetite, consistently poor sleep and aches around your body. When depression worsens, it could lead to contemplating suicide. Depressed people often feel that life is not worth living, but the intensity of depression varies from one person to another, as do the symptoms. The symptoms can include weight loss or weight gain, too much sleep or too little sleep, restlessness and agitation, slowed speech and movement, fatigue, guilt, difficulty concentrating, thoughts of suicide and death as well as attempting suicide.

The symptoms of depression can be ongoing, or they can manifest and leave to return later. They can also occur outside of the mind and can cause physical discomfort. Depression is not only emotional or mental. It could be physical too.

Signs of Depression at its Early Stages

At the onset of depression, some of the symptoms that we have pointed out in the preceding discussion would manifest. If not quickly diagnosed, these signs can pass for moodiness and can deteriorate. You must figure out soon if you will be developing depression. That way, you can quickly keep the situation under control. If you discover that you are having any of these signs and that it is persistent, it may be time for you to see a doctor.

Depression can begin with a change in your sleep routine which can include insomnia or sleeping for overly long periods. Other symptoms at the early stages include significant loss of interest in your daily routine and in activities that once gave you joy. Depression can make you uninterested in a way that your hobbies and social events can pass as a disturbance. You can also show a loss of sexual appetite. Depression can make you lose the ability to feel any form of joy or pleasure. So, it doesn't matter what activity is involved. You are simply not interested and genuinely do not enjoy them. You can also show high levels of anxiety as well as anger and irritability. Depressed individuals are often restless. They feel agitated and sometimes violent. Everything and everyone can be the loss of your irritation, and you begin to find that your tolerance levels are at an all-time low. You are also prone to a short temper.

Early signs of depression also include unintended weight gain or weight loss and appetite disorders. You suddenly eat too much or too little. At the early stages of depression, you can lose up to five percent of your weight in a month. Alternatively, you can gain weight even if you are not looking to. We can conclude that depression results in weight gain in some individuals because they become unmotivated to get moving and so lead a sedentary life within the period. You find that you may be eating too much or too little.

Another prominent sign of depression is fatigue. A depressed person can feel excessively weak and find that they have no energy to move through their day. It is often the case that they have exhausted their energy thinking. Overthinking is, therefore, one of the signs of depression. This can leave you feeling drained. If you were active before your depressive symptoms manifest, you could become sluggish as a result of the lack of energy. Even the little things you should do can become exhausting. In this way, depression causes you to spend a lot of time doing very little. You tend to move slowly through your day, find no joy in your activities and leave a lot of them undone.

When these symptoms of depression are overlooked, they tend to aggravate and usher in more prominent symptoms which in turn lead to significant depressive symptoms and an upturning of your life. Depression can feel very disorganizing and can give you the feeling that all the good in your life is gone. Don't give in to that lie.

Aggravated Symptoms of Depression

When the initial signs of depression are not treated, they can lead to further symptoms that deepen the condition. It is right for you to seek treatment early. It is also good for you to know what the aggravated symptoms are so that you know where your situation fits in the depression scale and what kind of remedy might be suitable for you.

The symptoms of depression that tell you that your situation is getting out of hand include feelings of helplessness or hopelessness, problems with concentration, self-loathing and physical pains and aches. You would start to feel like life is not worth living. You would think that there is nothing that can be done to make things better for you. These feelings will cause you to begin to hate yourself. Depression can make a person unable to focus.

For one thing, they have lost joy in pursuing their goals. Depressed people also have trouble making decisions when they get to this stage. Some people face problems with remembering things and have a general feeling of worthlessness and guilt. They see the mistakes around their lives as a fault of theirs. They can even begin to see themselves as having initiated the cause of the depression.

On a physical level, depression can cause you excessive discomforts like headaches, waist pain, stomach disorders and aching muscles. Depressed people are prone to escapist behavior. They also participate in compulsive behavior like gambling, substance abuse and reckless driving. Perhaps, the most worrying sign of depression is suicidal thoughts. Depression can put you at risk for suicide. If there is no reason to deal with the situation, that could be one. At its highest level, depression can make the individual that it torments to seek suicide as an escape from the pain, and the disturbing feelings of hopelessness and deep sadness. Such people can even become preoccupied with plans of dying. Some depressed people often begin to death clean and give their prized possessions away. They seem to have found the joy that they lost in death and the thought of death. In such circumstances, the depressed individual can become calm and happy because they think that they have found a solution to the menace that is depression. They are wrong. The proper path to take is to find the trail to that joy. Many people have found cannabis useful for helping them get back to normal.

Symptoms of depression can vary in men and women as well as in children. Let's take a look at how depression can manifest in different classes of people.

Depression Symptoms in Men

The American Psychological Association points out that around nine percent of men in the United States are undergoing depression and anxiety. Men are prone to alcohol misuse when they are depressed. They can also display excessive anger and take unnecessary risks. They are also likely to avoid their families and to run away from anything that puts them in a social situation. Depression can lead to overworking. They keep working without taking a break. We can say this is because they do not want to see anyone. Depression can cause men to be unable to perform their responsibilities both at work and at home. They also have tendencies of displaying abusive or controlling behavior. Often, this behavior is melted out on a spouse.

Depression Symptoms in Women

The Center for Disease Control and Prevention (CDC) has found depression to be nearly twice as common in women as it is in men. In the same regard, the symptoms that women exhibit is mostly different from those that men show. Women are more prone to mood swings. They get more fatigued than men who tend to work even harder. Women exhibit anxiety, irritability, fatigue and overthinking. They are often ruminating over negativity and assuring themselves of how bad things are and how they will only get worse. Some types of depression that affect women include premenstrual dysphoric disorder and postpartum depression.

Depression Symptoms in Children and Teens

It has been revealed by the Center for Disease Control and Prevention (CDC) that 3.2 percent of children and teens in the United States aged between three and seventeen have been diagnosed with depression. Children exhibit depression symptoms such as low energy, crying, clinginess, vocal outbursts and defiant behavior. Depending on the age of the child, they may not be able to tell you how they feel.

In teenagers, depression can be caused by puberty. They can start to feel sad as they try to get used to their physical changes. Depression can also result from peer pressure. Teens who are depressed will exhibit symptoms including withdrawal, feelings of guilt, helplessness and worthlessness, inability to concentrate and restlessness. They tend to avoid associating with or confiding in friends and family.

Depression Symptoms in College Students

The pressure that college brings with it can lead to depression. College students battle with different experiences and people all at once and are constantly in a state of trying to cope. Not all of them can handle the new level of exposure properly, and it is easy to find an outlet in depression. They begin to exhibit difficulty in concentrating on their academics; they develop irregular sleeping patterns, loss of appetite and withdrawal from social situations. Participating in activities that they once loved start to feel like a burden. As with everyone who goes through depression, college students experience high levels of sadness that often goes unexplained.

SHOULD YOU GET A PROFESSIONAL DIAGNOSIS?

Now that you have done a self-evaluation and you have figured out what the symptoms of depression are, the next thing to consider is whether you need a professional diagnosis. Like we have pointed out previously, many people do not know that they have depression until this is pointed out by a loved one. You may feel that your feelings of sadness are normal and that life is really as bad as you have concluded it to be. If your sad moods stay with you for weeks and months and would not be alleviated by other events occurring in your life, it is time to seek help. Also, you cannot diagnose yourself with depression, no matter how intense your symptoms are. Only your doctor can do that.

When you start to suspect that you may be suffering from depression, you should book an appointment with your doctor. Your doctor will combine several factors to determine if you have depression. Although how your doctor conducts the diagnosis is left to him, here are some of the things he is likely to take into consideration to determine whether or not you are depressed.

➢ **Physical Examination**

Sometimes, depression may be linked with a physical condition such as a visible health problem. Your doctor may conduct a physical exam and may take your medical history to determine whether you are depressed and whether you have the risks for it.

➢ **Laboratory Tests**

Your doctor is likely to carry out laboratory tests aimed at finding out if you have depression. He or she may take your blood samples and conduct tests on them. You may also have to undergo a thyroid test. The aim is to conduct a complete evaluation to see whether you have any medical symptoms of depression.

➢ Psychiatric Evaluation

Your doctor may refer you to a mental health professional or a psychiatrist to determine whether you have symptoms of depression. They may also find out whether the symptoms that you currently exhibit translate to depression. Your mental health professional will ask you questions relating to your thoughts and feelings and will evaluate your behavioral pattern before determining that you have depression.

➢ DSM-5

This refers to the Diagnostic and Statistical Manual of Mental Disorders. It is a manual published by the American Psychiatric Association, and it lists specific criteria for determining the presence of depression. Your mental health professional may use the standards contained in this manual to determine whether or not you are experiencing a depressive episode.

It can be challenging to decide that you need a professional diagnosis, but the moment you begin to wonder if you should, there is a high chance that you may be depressed. The right cause of action to take would be to book the appointment with your doctor and your mental health professional.

TYPES OF DEPRESSION

Depression is grouped into categories based on the symptoms exhibited. While some people experience brief episodes of depression, others have ongoing and often severe episodes. You cannot determine the type of depression that you have on your own. As with all things that concern this topic, you need your doctor to determine that. You need to undergo a proper diagnosis. You may suspect one or more types, but only your doctor can clarify the nature of depression that you have. A doctor may use what is called a specifier to show the kind of depression that you are going through. A specifier simply points to depression that is characterized by specific features. Depression is thus grouped along these lines.

In this section, we would learn about the types of depression, the specifiers, and how to spot each one. The two main types of depression are major depressive disorder and persistent disorder.

Major Depression

This can also be called major depressive disorder, and it is a severe kind of depression with symptoms that cannot leave on their own. Major depression can last up to six months at a time. This intensity is even much worse where it is left untreated. A person can encounter only one episode of depression in their lifetime. With major depression, this is often not the case. This kind of depression is often recurrent. It manifests as lack of pleasure in activities that you once enjoyed, excessive weight loss or weight gain, excessive sleep, fatigue, inability to concentrate, recurring thoughts of suicide or death, and so on.

For you to be diagnosed with major depression, you must have exhibited these symptoms for up to two weeks. Major depressive disorders have several subtypes, including anxious distress, seasonal patterns, atypical features, mixed features, psychotic features, catatonia, melancholic features, and peripartum onset. We will discuss these subtypes in the next section as they are characterized by specific features that are easily recognizable.

Persistent Depressive Disorder

This disorder is also called dysthymia. It is milder than major depression but is chronic. Unlike major depressive disorder, the symptoms of persistent depressive disorder must last up to two years. It includes low self-esteem, and medical experts assert that this form of depression can be treated successfully. However, you must stick to your treatment plan. This disorder can make it impossible for the person experiencing it to go about their normal activities. It is usually characterized by a disinterest in daily routine and an inability to enjoy life as one usually would.

How Depressed Are You?

Whether your depression is mild, acute or chronic will depend on which of the types you are going through. Knowing what kind of depression you have is essential to treating it. Your doctor would need to find out the specific depression that you are suffering to offer you the right treatment. This will also make it possible to manage symptoms. Perhaps, you also want to know how depressed you are. Depression is further categorized into the types discussed below.

Atypical Depression

Atypical depression is a variation of major depression. It has a specific symptom pattern and is a common subtype of major depression. Atypical depression manifests as temporary mood lifts and responds better to treatment. The symptom pattern of atypical depression is positive. The sufferer can undergo increased appetite and excessive sleep. He can feel happy when with friends and can gain unintended weight. The mood lifts do not, however, last long and a person suffering from atypical depression can be sensitive to rejection. Instead of exhibiting social withdrawal as is the case with some form of depression, he wants to be accepted. Atypical depression also manifests as a heavy feeling in the arms and legs.

Seasonal Affective Disorder (SAD)

This depression is seasonal. It occurs within the reduced daylight hours of winter. Seasonal Affective Disorder starts in winter and continues until spring. When the days get brighter, a person with Seasonal Affective Disorder also lightens in mood. This kind of depression is not very common and affects about two percent of people. A large part of these people are women and young persons.

If you have Seasonal Affective Disorder, you are bound to feel like you are a totally different person according to the seasons in a year. You can go from losing interests in activities that you love to having renewed interests in those activities when the season changes. During your depressed state, you will feel hopeless, stressed, nervous and sad. Your emotions will range from one of these to another. Seasonal Affective Disorder can also make you lose interest in your friends. When winter ends, you will go back to your former state and have renewed interest in your activities and your friends.

Dysthymia

Dysthymia is a chronic "low-grade" depression basically because it is recurrent and mild. Dysthymia includes brief periods of normal mood and can last for years. Also, Dysthymia can manifest minimal symptoms making it difficult to decipher. With Dysthymia, you can have low moods that are continuous, and you can quickly begin to believe that that is your normal mood. It is possible to experience other kinds of depression alongside Dysthymia, thereby undergoing double depression. What's more? Your other depressive episodes can be very major.

Depressive Specifiers

Specifiers are a kind of depression that have specific features. It is easy to decipher what you are going through from the features manifested. We will discuss more types of depression here that would help you spot if your mood shifts are something to worry about.

Psychotic Features

This kind of depression is accompanied by hallucinations or delusions that are centered around personal inadequacies and other negative things that the depressed person continues to ruminate about.

Mixed Features

This manifests as depression and mania occurring at the same time. The depressed individual will showcase symptoms that include increased energy, elevated self-esteem, and talking too much.

Atypical Features

This refers to atypical depression and includes symptoms such as temporary cheerfulness, sensitivity to rejection, increased appetite, excessive sleep and a heavy feeling in the arms and legs.

Anxious Distress

This kind of depression includes restlessness and anxiety. The depressed individual is always worried about future events and seems to have a loss of control.

Melancholic Features

This is a severe depression that manifests as finding no joy in things that once brought pleasure. It also includes terrible moods in the morning and waking up early, drastic change in appetite, feelings of guilt and agitation. A person with melancholic features will also become extremely sluggish.

Peripartum Onset

This kind of depression occurs during pregnancy. It also has a variation that is called postpartum depression and which occurs in the weeks and months that follow childbirth. The woman can become depressed and show deep sadness with no defined cause.

Catatonia

This depression manifests as motor activity. It involves purposeless or uncontrollable movement. It also includes fixed or inflexible posture. The person who has this depression will be restless and exhibit movement that is more than normal.

Depression can also be caused by other independent disorders. People who suffer from these disorders can also suffer from depression. These disorders can cause depression symptoms or can include depression as a symptom. In other words, if you have any of these disorders, you are at risk of depression. Sometimes, it could be that you are already depressed, and depression is a symptom of the disorder. It is important that you get an accurate diagnosis so that you can get the right treatment for you. If you have any of these disorders, your doctor should also check for the possibility of depression. We will discuss the disorders below.

Bipolar I and II disorders

This disorder is characterized by mood swings that move from highs to lows. A person with bipolar disorder would experience sharp mood swings and can shuffle between elevated moods to deep sadness. These characteristics make it difficult to differentiate this disorder from depression. Also, this disorder is capable of leading to depression. People who have bipolar disorder usually lose interest in their routine and in activities they once enjoyed. They often feel fatigued; have sleeping problems and sharp departures from their normal weight. They may also harbor thoughts of death or suicide. They also have difficulty remembering things. A person with bipolar disorder may experience one or more of these symptoms. With proper treatment, they can start to feel better and experience less of the symptoms.

Cyclothymic Disorder

This disorder is similar to bipolar disorder. It involves high and low moods which are a little milder than what a person with bipolar disorder will experience. The symptoms are also similar, and the condition can subside and rule out the possibility of deteriorating into depression.

Disruptive Mood Dysregulation Disorder

This is a mood disorder that is common in children. It manifests as chronic irritability and inflated anger that results in frequent and extreme temper outbursts. It is common for disruptive mood dysregulation disorder to develop into depressive disorder or anxiety disorder at the teenage years of the affected person or at early adulthood.

Premenstrual Dysphoric Disorder

This disorder is found in women. It involves hormonal changes that begin a week before a woman's menstrual cycle and gets better once her flow begins. Usually, as her period comes to an end, the symptoms associated with premenstrual dysphoric disorder also end. This disorder can make the woman excessively sad and highly irritable within the period and can deteriorate into depression if not properly treated.

It is important to note that behavioral patterns and lifestyle influences, such as substance abuse can lead to depression. Similarly, medications can cause depression as a side effect, even where such medication was prescribed. There are also medical conditions that could lead to depression. To rule out this later cause, a doctor would usually take your medical history and conduct tests aimed at ensuring that your depression is not rooted in illnesses of another kind. Where it is, this medical condition will be treated accordingly. Where it is not, you will be offered other treatment options. As we will see in later parts of this book, cannabis is a useful treatment tool for depression.

WHEN DEPRESSION GETS COMPLICATED

While it is difficult to contend with depression as a regular person, it is even more difficult to deal with depression under certain circumstances. Depression can make otherwise seemingly complicated conditions much worse. Instead of dealing with one problem, when depression enters the picture, you have to deal with two. Even if it were a positive condition you were dealing with, such as pregnancy, depression could make it tougher. Let's take a look at how you can prevent depression and how depression can be complicated by other medical conditions.

Testing for Depression

It is essential to point out here that there is no single test for depression. When you go to your doctor for treatment of depression, he would first need to put you through a diagnosis to confirm whether you have the condition. He would do this through an evaluation of your symptoms and may refer you for psychological evaluation. Your doctor will ask you a lot of questions relating to your moods, your sleeping patterns, appetite, enthusiasm and thought processes. It is advisable to be as ready as you can before you see your doctor. This would make the evaluation process much easier. We will go into details of how you should prepare for your meeting with your doctor in chapter six of this book.

Depression test may also include a physical exam and blood tests. Some of the health problems that a physical exam can bring to light include vitamin D deficiency and thyroid problems. Depression can get worse if it is left untreated and can result in complications such as panic attacks, social isolation, self-harm, problems with your relationships, and so on. It is essential to go for a depression test to avoid all these states and even much worse complications.

You would usually not be diagnosed with depression if your symptoms do not last up to two weeks. Your depressive episode must have occurred for two weeks or longer and must include at least five known symptoms of depression.

Do You Have to be Hospitalized?

In extreme cases of depression, you may be required to stay back at the hospital. Where you are experiencing suicidal thoughts, taking unusual risks or exhibiting tendencies to harm yourself and others, your primary care doctor might recommend a hospital stay. In other cases, partial hospitalization or day treatment programs may be enough to boost your mood. Adequate counseling support has been integrated into these programs to help ease your symptoms.

DEPRESSION AND ANXIETY

Even though anxiety can occur on its own, like stress, it can become intermingled with depression. A person who has depression may also have anxiety. The two conditions can occur simultaneously. Medical experts assert that over seventy percent of people who are depressed have symptoms of anxiety. It is, therefore, common to treat depression and anxiety together. The two conditions have different causes, but they share similar symptoms including irritability, problems with sleep, inability to concentrate or to recollect things, and so on. The treatment regimen of depression and anxiety is mostly similar. A doctor can verify whether both conditions coexist and can work out the treatment plan that is suitable for you.

Depression and anxiety coexist because it is so common for one mental health condition to lead to another. About forty-five percent of people who have one mental health problem often end up diagnosed with another. In one peculiar study, researchers found that half of the people who have depression also have anxiety. The root cause of anxiety and depression are different, but they share similar symptoms. They can also be treated through the same procedure.

Anxiety is commonly associated with anticipation. When you are expecting a big day, you can feel anxious about it. At what point then does it become a mental health illness? Chronic anxiety involves feeling fatigued, problems with sleep, grinding your teeth, racing heart, muscle tension, inability to concentrate, and so on. You will notice that some of these symptoms are also symptoms of anxiety. This kind of anxiety impedes the thoughts and causes fear that makes daily activities almost impossible to navigate. A person with chronic anxiety would also experience restlessness, panic, dread, irritability and other emotional highs.

MANAGING DEPRESSION AND ANXIETY

The symptoms characterizing both depression and anxiety is such that deviate from our normal experience. They intend to impose a new normal. However, self-evaluation can help you spot the changes quickly. If you start to feel different or exhibit behaviors that are new and indicative of these conditions, you should not hesitate to seek the help of a healthcare provider. Depression and anxiety are highly treatable if they are spotted early. Only you can spot it early. If you wait until somebody tells you that you are depressed, chances are that the situation has already deteriorated or at least has become pronounced. In some cases, this can make treatment more difficult than it should be.

You can find self-diagnosis tests online from medical websites. This will help you stay on top of the situation and decipher what is happening to you before it is too late. Note that these tests are only a preparation for your actual meeting with a doctor or other healthcare professional. Similarly, there are a few self-care tips that can help you deal with depression. These self-care tips carry different outcomes for different people going through depression and anxiety and in some cases; they may not yield the desired result.

➢ Let Your Feelings Find Expression

Yes, it may not be a good feeling, but it's occurring anyway. Allow yourself to feel all those emotions. Remind yourself often that this is not your fault and it is not happening because of some deficiency that you have. Depression and anxiety are not a result of weakness, and so they should not be something to be ashamed of. They are medical conditions for which you should seek proper medical help. You are feeling the way that you feel because your triggers are finding expression and not because you did something wrong.

➢ Engage in Physical Activity

Whether it is making your bed, taking out the trash or going for a walk, make sure that you are always active. Physical activity can take your mind off the things that are worrying to you. They can also help you feel that you have control over something. Shift your perspective from those nagging feelings that you cannot control and give your life some form of order. Carry out tasks that you can complete and allow yourself feel like you have accomplished something. This can help to push the feelings of hopelessness and sadness away.

> **Create a Routine**

It is possible for your life to feel completely out of order. Creating a routine can help you manage that, especially during this trying time. Having a sense of order in your day can make your life feel like it still belongs to you. Routines can help ease both depression and anxiety as they give you a sense of structure and reduce symptoms.

> **Tend to your Taste Buds**

At least once a week, eat something nutritious, and that can awaken your senses. Foods like apples, nuts and pasta can quickly comfort you and elevate your mood. They may not be nutritious though, so do not take them all day long. Instead, combine them with other nutrient-dense foods like fruits and vegetables. They will awaken your senses and push both depression and anxiety away.

➢ Maintain A Sleep Routine

Both disorders can tamper with your sleep. With both depression and anxiety, it is easy to sleep too little or not at all. Consciously create a sleep schedule that you adhere to. You can choose to sleep at specific times in your day. You can choose to sleep early. Make sure that you are getting the recommended seven to eight hours a day. Sleep has a way of pushing away so many medically inclined woes so make it a priority. Poor sleep is associated with other medical problems like endocrine trouble, cardiovascular and immune symptoms, among others.

➢ Engage in an Activity that you Enjoy

Depression and anxiety can make you begin to lose your joy in activities that you once couldn't do without. These activities can cheer you up. So, now that you do not want to do them is precisely the time to do them. Get active and shake off the sad moods. These activities could include watching TV, listening to music, playing sports and so on. Go on and do them!

➢ Talk to Someone

Sometimes, all it takes to keep depression and anxiety symptoms from worsening is to talk about them. Reach out to someone that you trust and tell them what you are going through. Make sure you are talking to somebody that you are comfortable with, as this will enable you to show how you truly feel.

> ### Do Something Soothing

When you are depressed or anxious, there is a high tendency of you staying indoors. This can only worsen your symptoms. So, get out there and do something that will soothe your nerves. You can go for a massage or join a yoga class. Your options are only limited by your imagination. Think of something you have always wanted to do and do it!

If you try all of these and your symptoms only worsen, it may be time to see your doctor. Remember that with the right amount of effort, you can kick out depression and anxiety. Your doctor may recommend cannabis for helping ease the symptoms of both anxiety and depression. Interestingly also, cannabis can be used to ease stress. It is able to do this by removing or reducing the cause of stress.

DEPRESSION AND OBSESSIVE-COMPULSIVE DISORDER (OCD)

Anxiety is so commonly associated with depression that it has further complications. One type of anxiety disorder that occurs during depression is what is known as obsessive-compulsive disorder. This disorder manifests as obsessions. It ignites unwanted and often repeated thoughts, fears and urges. These obsessions cause a strain then leads to compulsions which evidence you behaving in ways that you think will make you feel better. The critical thing about this disorder is that both the obsessions and compulsions happen at a repeated rate. Also, it is quickly followed by withdrawal symptoms in which case you feel isolated and begin to detach from your friends and family. You begin to participate less in social situations that you once enjoyed. It is this withdrawal that increases your risk for and eventually leads to depression.

The result is that it is quite common for somebody who has obsessive-compulsive disorder to also have depression. In fact, the number of people who have both obsessive-compulsive disorder and depression is placed at a high eighty percent. Even worse is the fact that if you have one anxiety disorder, you are prone to developing another. The combination of these two disorders is a concern in children. They can begin to exhibit OCD at a very young age and develop depression as a result. You must watch your children carefully for any signs of withdrawal from their friends. The child may feel less special, isolated and may eventually begin to avoid social situations.

DEPRESSION AND PSYCHOSIS

It is possible to suffer from a mental condition called psychosis if you are diagnosed with major depression. Although this is not the case for everyone, the National Alliance on Mental Illness (NAMI) have estimated that up to twenty percent of people who were diagnosed with major depression also have psychotic symptoms. In such situations, a person is said to be suffering from depressive psychosis. Depressive psychosis occurs when a person has major depression and psychotic symptoms. He feels sad and lacks the energy to carry out everyday activity. On top of this, he experiences paranoia, delusions and hallucinations.

The condition is known by other names including delusional depression, psychotic depression, major depressive disorder with mood-congruent psychotic features and major depressive disorder with mood-incongruent features.

A person who has depressive psychosis experiences hallucination alongside the usual symptoms of depression, such as deep sadness. They see and hear things that do not exist. Depressive psychosis is a hazardous mental health condition as it takes the sufferer through feelings of hopelessness, sadness and irritability that eventually translates to thoughts of suicide and taking unfathomable risks.

Medical experts are unable to explain why depression and psychosis occur together. Although the condition has no known cause, some people in the medical community think that it is a result of chemical imbalances in the brain. But this is only a speculation as research has not identified a cause. In spite of this, they have been able to develop effective treatment procedures for both conditions.

It is believed that depressive psychosis may be genetically linked. Researchers are yet to figure out the specific gene that causes the problem. However, studies show that if you have a close family member who has the condition, you stand at a higher risk of getting it too. Similarly, women experience depressive psychosis much more than men. It was pointed out in the journal, BMC Psychiatry that older adults were at great risks for psychotic depression.

To enable your doctor to diagnose you correctly, you have to open up during your evaluation and let your treatment team know all about what you are going through. It is easy to shy away from telling them what you go through, especially where you have psychotic symptoms, but this will only make your doctor give you a wrong diagnosis. This can also affect your treatment and your overall recovery. In addition to the known signs of depression, people who have depressive psychosis will also experience psychotic symptoms. Also, these symptoms would have lasted for two weeks or more. Make sure that you are giving your doctor the full picture of what is happening to you. This will save you both a lot of trouble. If you have depressive psychosis, you are likely to hold false beliefs combined with feelings of guilt. You may think that something which is happening to your body is your fault and is a punishment. In reality, the beliefs that you hold when you have depressive psychosis would not be true at all. If you feel that you are delusional and are hallucinating, you should see your doctor immediately.

DEPRESSION IN PREGNANCY

We have pointed out elsewhere in this book that even positive experiences can trigger depression in some cases. While pregnancy is an exciting time for a woman and her family, it is possible for her to become depressed. In fact, it is quite common. When a pregnant woman is depressed, she will exhibit symptoms such as anxiety, persistent feelings of hopelessness and sadness, inability to concentrate, changes in appetite, a departure from her eating habits, difficulty sleeping or a change in her sleeping patterns, and frequent thoughts of death or suicide. Simply put, she will manifest the symptoms of depression that we have discussed in this book.

A pregnant woman needs to seek an appointment with her doctor if any of these feelings linger for two weeks or more. All the treatment options for depression can only be used during pregnancy with medical supervision. Similarly, a pregnant or breastfeeding mother should not use cannabis without discussing it with her doctor. It has been found that cannabis is capable of stunting the child's development during pregnancy and affecting the baby's health.

Depression Treatment Options

You need to know the treatment options that are available to you. The treatment regimen that your doctor and your mental health professional will prescribe is mainly dependent on your symptoms and their severity. It becomes vital then that you visit a healthcare professional as soon as your symptoms manifest.

Additionally, medications designed to cure depression do not do that. What antidepressants can do for you is to correct the underlying chemical imbalance that causes the situation. Even so, they are known to do this only while you are taking them. A depressive episode may pass eventually, but this does not point to a cure. Some of your depression triggers may never go anywhere. As a mental health expert puts it, they are only waiting for 'the right set of circumstances.' It behoves on you then to put the situation under control at all times.

The results of leaving depression untreated are debilitating, and it is impossible to have a routine if the mental illness is not taken care of. Depression can affect every part of your life if you do not treat it. Chronic depression is dangerous because it can lead to thoughts of suicide. It can make the person involved to take unfathomable and unrealistic risks. Who is to say that eventual suicide may not be one of these? Depression can make its victim to harbor thoughts of death always and to find pleasure in such thoughts because they see them as a relief. If left unattended to, the consequences are always tragic.

In the pages that follow, we would be discussing the treatment options available to you and providing a guide to help you understand what you should look out for in your treatment regimen. Your doctor will give you the best treatment option for your condition. You must provide him with as much information as is available to you as this will make the process of your diagnosis easy, and you will get an accurate treatment plan. A treatment regimen that does not suit your full symptoms will only make you regress. Be as truthful as you can be. Otherwise, your treatment team can miss out on additional disorders that you might be experiencing. In that case, your prescribed treatment would not adequately address your situation and any improvements you experience would be slow.

Before you meet with your doctor, get a good grasp of your symptoms and get in touch with your feelings. You do not want to miss out on any of the details. Your evaluation will take the form of a series of questions. Being able to answer accurately will lead to a proper diagnosis and in turn, an adequate treatment prescription. Preparing beforehand tends to make the evaluation more efficient, thereby allowing the time to focus on an in-depth analysis of your situation. Similarly, you would be able to venture into topics that worry you. The evaluation process with your doctor and with your mental health professional provides you with an opportunity to have an honest discussion about what you have been going through and to get the help that you need.

Let's take a look at some of the questions that your doctor may ask you during evaluation. You can jot this down in a journal and try providing accurate answers before you go for your appointment. This will get rid of the possibility of guessing what your answers should be and providing your doctor with inaccurate information. Pick a paper and pen and figure out how these questions relate to you!

- When did you start noticing your symptoms?

- How long have you been depressed?

- Do you find it challenging to go through with your daily activities as usual?

- Do you have a family member that has suffered from depression in the past?

- Do you often think about suicide and death?

- Do you go from feeling alive and happy to feeling down without notice?

- Do you take alcohol or drugs?

- Do you have any other health problem, whether physical or mental?

What you should be expecting during your evaluation includes questions about your symptoms, medications that you have taken in the past and your personal information, including significant life changes that you have recently gone through. Now that you are prepared to give adequate information to help with your diagnosis, you should prepare your concerns and get ready to have your doctor or mental health professional answer them. You may write down your questions, or you may go with a loved one who would serve to remind you of anything you may have forgotten.

There is a broad range of treatment options, all of which we would discuss in this chapter. Medication and psychotherapy are two of the most effective and immediate. While medication can instantly relieve your symptoms, psychotherapy works to walk you through your feelings and ensure that you come out healthy on the other side. It is, therefore, possible to take both treatment options together. In some cases, medication alone can improve your symptoms. But it must be combined with proper self-care. Whatever treatment option you choose, taking care of yourself is key to overcoming depression.

Where these two treatment options are not effecting a relief, your doctor or mental health professional may prescribe other advanced or alternative treatment plans. The key to making your treatment work is sticking to it and checking your progress with your doctor. In severe situations, you may need a hospital stay, or you may be required to participate in an outpatient treatment program. If you are given these options, you have to stick to them until your symptoms improve.

MEDICATION

Medications are prescribed to deal with the chemical imbalance in the brain that is associated with depression. Medication as a treatment option for depression is widely advertised, but that doesn't make it the most effective. The treatment plan that is suitable for you will largely depend on your symptoms. These symptoms surpass chemical imbalances in the brain, and some of them may be emotional. Medication can relieve some of your symptoms, especially if what you are going through is moderate or severe depression. Medication is not a long-term solution as it does not cure depression, but it can make you feel better, and it can improve your symptoms. Depression medications are called antidepressants, and they come with side effects. Also, withdrawing from the medication can pose a problem. As a result, the Food and Drug Administration (FDA) has placed a strict stipulation on the distribution of antidepressants. These standards require that all antidepressants carry a black box warning. This is the strictest warning for all prescriptions. If you decide to use medications, you should also follow the other treatment regimen prescribed for you. Make appropriate lifestyle changes that can prevent a reoccurrence.

Depression medication includes tricyclic antidepressants, monoamine oxidase inhibitors (MAOIs), atypical antidepressants, and so on. Your doctor may prescribe other medications for you to add to an antidepressant. Depending on your type of depression, you may also be asked to combine two antidepressants or to add medications like antipsychotics, anti-anxiety or mood stabilizers. The medication you are adding to your antidepressant may be taken only for a short time. Make sure that you ask your doctor for full details on how to use medication for depression and which ones are recommended for you.

Genetics may play a role in depression and how you react to medication. An antidepressant might be useful for you if it was effective in treating a family member. You may also try several medications before you find one that works for you. It can feel like a tedious process, but you need to push yourself to get it done. The effects of medication are not instant. You may need to wait for weeks to see whether your symptoms improve. Your body would be trying to adjust within the time before it allows the medication to take full effect — several factors, including genetics, influence how your body responds to medication.

Withdrawal symptoms often follow when you stop taking a depression medication abruptly. You should speak to your doctor and receive a go-ahead before you stop taking an antidepressant. This is also the case when you miss your doses. You can worsen your symptoms instead of improving them. Your doctor can work out a plan with you that will help you reduce your doses one step at a time and ensure that you do not suffer from depression symptoms. You must never take a medication that is not prescribed by your doctor. Before using an antidepressant, ensure that it is something prescribed by your doctor and that you are clear about how to use it.

The fact that your symptoms have improved is not enough reason to stop taking your medication. This will lead to a reoccurrence and relapse. If you are unsure about an antidepressant or other prescription, let your doctor know. If you want to stop taking a medication, maybe because it gives you some form of discomfort, discuss this with your doctor as well. The side effects of antidepressants include nausea, diarrhea, low blood sugar, constipation, sexual dysfunction and weight loss. You may also notice an unusual rash. In severe cases, medications can increase suicidal thoughts in children, teens and young adults under twenty-five at the beginning months of the treatment. A good antidepressant will have these side effects listed on the packaging.

It becomes important that you do not isolate yourself when you are taking antidepressants. You need close monitoring from your loved ones to ensure that your symptoms are not worsening. It is usual to experience behavioral change when you are starting a new medication or taking a different dosage. If suicidal thoughts arise during the use of an antidepressant, you should get help immediately. You will need to see your doctor to enable you to take appropriate actions for your situation. When the suicidal thoughts pass, medication can reduce suicide risk and improve your depression symptoms by boosting your mood.

PSYCHOTHERAPY

Psychotherapy is a treatment regimen for depression that involves talking about your condition with a mental health professional. Psychotherapy is also called talk therapy or psychological therapy. Although there are different types of psychotherapy, the most effective for depression are cognitive behavioral therapy (CBT) and interpersonal therapy.

Psychotherapy helps ease depression symptoms by walking you through the emotional dynamics of the situation. The treatment can help you adjust your thinking, beliefs and behaviors in a way that improves your symptoms. They can help you adapt to challenging situations that you may be going through. Psychotherapy can enhance your relationships, your problem-solving skills and help you set better goals. When you are depressed, you might be unable to manage expectations. Through psychotherapy, your therapist can help you realize that your goals may be unrealistic, and there may be a better way to get things done. Psychotherapy is intended to help you cope, and your sessions with your therapist can help you gain control over your life. Your interactions with yourself and with others will be much more positive and beneficial to everyone involved. This way, you can let go of the negative and allow positives to influence your everyday life.

In some cases, psychotherapy may be your very first prescribed treatment. For some other people, they may have to combine both psychotherapy and medication. Psychotherapy is excellent for situations where there is no underlying medical cause for the depressive symptoms. Your therapist will help you feel better and teach you what you need to know to avoid a reoccurrence. The essence of psychotherapy is that you can overcome depression by enhancing your thinking and learning appropriate behavioral skills. You will learn what the actual cause of your depression is and be equipped to avoid your triggers. Through psychotherapy, you will be able to detach from what you are feeling and make the changes necessary for a healthy life. If unhealthy relationships surround you, your psychotherapy session can help you see that, and it can help you to build healthier relationships and avoid social isolation. For some of us, the reason for our depression relapses is the fact that we are overwhelmed, and we keep on taking more. Psychotherapy will show you how to set healthy boundaries. Your talk therapy session can help you identify which boundaries are necessary, and when you follow through on them, you will relieve stress. Remember that stress is a pivotal depression trigger in its chronic state. Perhaps, the best part of psychotherapy is that it provides you with an opportunity to walk through your problems with a trusted friend who can listen objectively and without judgment. You are also able to get feedback that allows you to move forward in your life.

Should You Go For An Individual Or Group Therapy?

Depression therapy can be one-on-one, or it may be conducted in a group. Whatever mode of therapy you choose or that is recommended for you is as great as the other. In a group therapy, you get to meet and interact with people who have similar problems as you. Therapy sessions last for about an hour in each case and can run multiple times within a year.

You may not see the results of therapy immediately, but it will eventually get better. You need to develop the tenacity to keep at it by preparing your mind for what is ahead. Be honest with your therapist as this will make for progress with your evaluation and will also make sure that your diagnosis is correct. While both individual and group therapy are great for coping with depression, both have their distinct features and usefulness. Individual therapy will allow you to build a solid relationship with your therapist. You will also feel more disposed to sharing sensitive information. When you are in a group, you are likely to be more protective of some of your feelings and experiences, and this will not help recovery. Along this line, listening to other people and realizing that you are not the only one going through this can strengthen your resolve and help you heal faster. Experts have suggested that this can also build your self-esteem. Perhaps, what is best about group therapy is that there is a mixture of experiences available. You will find strength in the experiences that are shared and will realize too that you are moving. This sense of control over the situation is vital to overcoming depression. Social isolation can be quickly replaced with a support network of people who understand what you are going through. With psychotherapy, it will get worse before it gets better. Yet, you will be astonished at how close to cure you are.

When you are choosing your therapist, make sure that you select somebody that you connect with. This is important to succeeding with your therapy sessions. You want to work with someone who is supportive of you and who will work with you to help you overcome depression. Choosing the wrong therapist can invalidate the whole process and even make you feel worse off than when you began. If you are already working with a therapist that you do not connect with or if you start to feel that this may not be right, it is time for you to find someone new. You should be bold enough to seek something that works better for you and that moves you forward to recovery instead of backward to your depressive symptoms. Therapy can be great and effective only if you have a trusting relationship in place.

It may feel difficult to find a therapist, but with a guide on where to look, the process can get easier. You can get recommendations on where to find a good therapist from your friends, family and social circle. Remember that depression is not something to be ashamed of, and you should not feel bad about asking for help. Your doctor can also recommend a good therapist to you. National Mental Health Organizations have a pool of licensed therapists from which you can get a referral. Community health clinics and religious organizations are also great places to get referrals at a minimal cost.

There are alternative therapy formats like online sessions over smart devices, relaxation techniques and herbal supplements. Treating with cannabis can also come into the picture. Cannabis has proven useful for making depressive symptoms and other associated mental health conditions feel better. Patients can find respite from a treatment program that uses cannabis. Before you begin your treatment, it is important to discuss the alternatives with your primary care doctor.

COGNITIVE BEHAVIORAL THERAPY

Cognitive behavioral therapy is popularly used to treat depression and deserves a separate section in this book. The treatment method operates by opening you up to your thoughts and carrying you through the process of replacing unhealthy thought patterns. Cognitive behavioral therapy is a talk therapy, and it is as good as medication in treating depression. In some cases, cognitive behavioral therapy could do a better job than medication. However, the treatment option is effective for mild and moderate depression. In chronic cases, cognitive behavioral therapy alone will not be enough to treat depression. However, if you are working with a highly skilled therapist, it would make symptoms of severe depression more manageable. CBT is also very effective when you combine it with medication.

What your therapist does during your sessions is to help you identify your negative thoughts, including ways that you have been lying to yourself. He then helps you to replace this with a healthier thought pattern by making you set more realistic goals. An example is depression caused by feelings of guilt. You think that your life will only go in the wrong direction and you concentrate on your flaws. Your therapist can help you see everything that is good in your life and show you that you are not altogether weak. Through cognitive behavioral therapy, you can become more self-aware. You will realize what your negative thought patterns are, and you will learn how to replace them with positive thoughts. CBT helps you to put in the effort each day to try again. It pushes you to get up and try again. By replacing the thoughts that make you feel that life is altogether hopeless, you are about to live a healthier, more fulfilled life.

For CBT to work correctly, you have to let your therapist know what you are thinking and how you are feeling. Your therapist will help you see that those thoughts are false and negative. He will then take you through getting rid of them by exchanging them for more positive and realistic thoughts. If you recognize that you are not the cause of your problems and that things will improve, you are steps closer to overcoming depression.

Mental health professionals that offer CBT sessions include psychologists, licensed clinical social workers, licensed counselors, and so on. The sessions include individual and group therapies, but you can opt for self-help or online therapy sessions. The sessions are between ten to twenty, depending on your progress and your treatment goals. Your therapist will help you with setting treatment goals. In severe cases, therapy can last up to a year and go beyond that time frame. You will learn skills for preventing relapse, and your therapist will monitor your progress, including whether treatment goals are getting achieved. It is essential that you select your therapy carefully. You can choose from a pool of licensed professionals. Make sure that your therapist is licensed and certified and that he works within the areas that you need help with. Do not be afraid to open up to your therapist, and if you feel uncomfortable, you may need someone new.

BRAIN STIMULATION

Where these treatment options do not ease your depression symptoms, you may be taken through the medical alternatives. Depression can be medically corrected through brain stimulation which includes transcranial magnetic stimulation and electroconvulsive therapy. For ease of understanding, we would only explain transcranial magnetic stimulation in this book. The aim of brain stimulation is to trigger the mood cells in the brain and by so doing make you feel better.

Transcranial Magnetic Stimulation

In some cases, major depression may resist treatment. If your depression is not responding to medication, therapy and self-care, you can choose to go for transcranial magnetic stimulation. This treatment option is a noninvasive procedure that directs electromagnetic energy to the nerve cells of the brain that regulate mood. The recurring energy currents enter the skull through a treatment coil that is placed against the scalp, and the patient doesn't feel any pain. This works to improve the interchange of signals between parts of the brain in a way that eases depression symptoms. If your depression is treatment-resistant, transcranial magnetic stimulation can lead to relief. However, it does not lead to a cure. You will experience an improved level of energy, and the procedure can give you the drive you need to make the necessary lifestyle changes. Your doctor may also decide to use transcranial magnetic stimulation which uses a battery-operated stimulator instead of an electromagnetic coil. Discuss the options with your doctor to know which one suit you best.

SELF CARE

Taking good care of you is a pivotal part of overcoming depression. In some cases, you may not need any other form of treatment. No matter what treatment regimen you are on, making the right lifestyle changes can make your symptoms ease faster. Effecting changes to your routine and pushing yourself out of the redundancy that characterizes depression can help you heal more quickly. Challenge yourself to try something new. You would be inactive most of the time, but this will only worsen your symptoms. Do something you have always wanted to do. Go somewhere new. Force yourself to enjoy new activities. Get up and begin to plan activities that you would love. Depression will not leave on its own without any effort on your part. Instead, it would get much worse. Consistently look for new activities that can pull you out of your moods. Do not isolate yourself from your friends as this will only worsen your symptoms. If you find that you have forgotten how to have fun, you should start learning it all over again.

Other self-care tips for overcoming depression include exercising regularly, eating well, getting enough sleep and having a strong support network. Exercise can increase brain chemicals that ease depression. You may need to put in the extra effort like working out a meal plan, a sleep routine, and an exercise regimen to help make the adjusting process easier. Always choose a less stressful alternative. Depression is more likely to ease when you take care of yourself than when you don't. Substance abuse and alcohol misuse are known to worsen depression, so you may want to let those go as well.

Journaling is an important habit that you should inculcate when you are battling depression. Writing things done has a tendency of relieving us of whatever pressure we feel. Create a journal and put down things that you are thankful for. Read this whenever you feel sad. You should also write down your feelings. Doing this will help yours to trace the patterns that you exhibit more easily and will also help you to figure out what your depression triggers are. Other outlets that are similar to this for managing depression include reading, watching TV and listening to music. Make sure that what you listen to or read is something that is motivating. Avoid sad themes as these can take you back to your depressive state.

DEALING WITH THE STRESS AND DEPRESSION DYNAMIC

Stress impacts profoundly on depression because people who are stressed are more likely to conduct themselves in a way that eventually affects their moods negatively. They are prone to developing unhealthy patterns of behavior which can lead to depression. If you are undergoing a high level of stress, you should effect the lifestyle changes discussed in this book to make the situation better and to prevent or ease depression. You should also consider including cannabis in your treatment regimen.

TREATMENT FOR DEPRESSION IN PREGNANCY

Depression during pregnancy usually occurs in up to eighty percent of mothers between one to two weeks after childbirth. This kind of depression is called postpartum depression. Mothers with postpartum depression often feel detached from their babies and have no sense of joy from delivery. The symptoms range from feelings of sadness to exhaustion and loss of appetite. As with other kinds of depression, postpartum depression can be treated by medication and therapy. Your doctor can recommend one or both treatment methods. You must also consciously make lifestyle changes that are geared towards helping you recover. You may not find a treatment plan that works for you immediately, but when you try a little more, you can work out something alongside your doctor that makes your symptoms better.

If you do not see improvements immediately, do not stop taking your prescribed antidepressants. They will eventually lighten your mood, but your body needs a little bit of time to adjust. You may feel fatigued while you are taking antidepressants, but this shouldn't discourage you. The side effects of medication will soon pass. Make sure you verify that it is safe to take the antidepressant in question. Some medication may not be suitable for you while you are breastfeeding. Let your doctor know that you will be breastfeeding. This will help him to recommend medication that suits you better.

Your primary care doctor may refer you to a mental health professional for further evaluation. During therapy, you will be able to get the help you need, including counselling to overcome depression. Your therapist will help you through your symptoms and provide you with strategies for healing. Take care of yourself. Do less than you usually would. Let the people around you know that you need some support and pay attention to yourself. Be careful not to withdraw or isolate yourself. You can also join a support group that addresses the needs of people like you. If you are going through postpartum depression, you might experience these depressive symptoms for six months or longer. With the right treatment, your symptoms will subside within this time. There are also natural remedies and supplements available to treat postpartum, but you must check in with your doctor before you try any medication. Although cannabis is a natural remedy and supplements in many of its forms, it may not be recommended for treating depression, stress or anxiety in pregnant women and breastfeeding mothers.

Treating Depression and Anxiety

Your doctor may put you through a combination of physical examination and screening tests to determine whether you have depression and anxiety. Like some of the symptoms, depression and anxiety can use the same treatment methods. You may need to undergo therapy or to take medications to help ease your symptoms. You may be given an antidepressant, anti-anxiety medications and mood stabilizers. You may also have to go through a cognitive behavioral therapy, interpersonal therapy or another form of therapy that your doctor thinks is best for you. Make sure you let your doctor know before you try any alternative forms of therapy.

Treatment for Depressive Psychosis

Although the Food and Drug Administration (FDA) is yet to approve a treatment method for depressive psychosis, the two overlapping conditions can be treated separately. There are two treatment options for depressive psychosis which are medication and electroconvulsive therapy (ECT). You may be given both antidepressants and antipsychotics to help adjust the hormonal imbalance in the brain. The medications include selective serotonin reuptake inhibitors (SSRIs), atypical antipsychotics, and so on. Cannabis topicals, sprays and pills that are made with CBD are effective antipsychotics medication that can effectively treat psychosis. What we have done with the clinical conditions is an extensive exposition on them and all the possible medical treatments applicable. Medicinal cannabis as we have seen is a very crucial treatment method for all these conditions.

Electroconvulsive therapy is believed to be able to ease psychotic symptoms where it involves suicidal thoughts and to make you feel better. You may also be given medications to take after ECT. The side effects of the treatment for depressive psychosis include short term memory loss, weight gain or weight loss, drowsiness, dizziness and changes in sleeping patterns. You can take psychotherapy to help you, walk through your fears and learn how to deal with a relapse.

Clinical Uses of Cannabis for Depression, Anxiety and Stress

As we have seen through the discourse, cannabis is great for treating depression, anxiety and stress. In fact, the relief that it offers is almost instant. Subsequently, we will see how easing these conditions automatically make insomnia find its way and corrects other sleep disorders. Cannabis also treats post-traumatic stress disorder effectively and this is also a condition that can occur alongside any of these clinical conditions. It would appear therefore that cannabis is useful for treating a lot of clinical conditions occurring at the same time.

A recent research has ventured into the efficacy of cannabis to combat depression, anxiety and stress. The results showed that by inhaling cannabis, participants were able to reduce depressive symptoms by up to eighty-nine percent. Anxiety, on the other hand, was reduced by ninety-three percent with the same results indicated for stress. It appears that cannabis is as soothing as can be.

The study went further to see how taking cannabis can affect the different sexes and if there was a correlation. Researchers found that women experienced a greater reduction in anxiety symptoms than men did. Also important is the fact that participants recorded a reduction in depressive symptoms where the amount of CBD was higher than THC. For anxiety however, the study was unable to show the specific interaction between THC and CBD. Researchers were unable to show which of these cannabinoids were responsible for the improvements of the anxiety symptoms in the participants.

In combating stress, it was shown that there was a significant interaction between THC and CBD. Stress was reduced in participants at a higher level when the dose of THC and CBD was almost equal. In fact where the strain showed differences in the THC and CBD ratio, there was almost no change in the symptoms. The higher both cannabinoids are in the dose of medicinal cannabis given to the patient, the more likely that he would experience a reduction in his stress symptoms.

This study, like many others, shows that medicinal cannabis is helpful in dissuading the symptoms and effects of mental health conditions. It is also great for helping patients who have the conditions find relief.

Chronic Pain

We have seen that depression, anxiety and stress can get intertwined. Regardless of how complicated the situation gets, cannabis is an effective treatment tool for each condition. Medicinal cannabis can be used to treat depression, anxiety and stress whether these conditions occur together or separately. Throughout this book, we have emphasized that the most popular use for medicinal cannabis is chronic pain.

Severe pain is a clinical condition and a symptom for several other conditions. Cannabis has been used by experts to make patients who have chronic pain feel better. Cannabis is effective for treating neuropathic pain. When patients suffer from pain that other potent pain medications are unable to relieve, cannabis can quickly come to the rescue to make the situation better. In fact, medical practitioners are agreed that combining cannabis with another medication can increase the potency of that medication. It can also result in a reduction of the appropriate dosage for that medication. If a patient is being administered opiod for example, adding cannabis to this will mean that he will take a lower dose of opiod. The cannabis content of the medication offered will also increase the potency of opiod. Cannabis has been used to relieve patients of otherwise unbearable pain. It is also used to relieve pain at the end of life.

It can be consumed by applying it directly to the affected area and it can be inhaled by smoking or as a pile. Cannabinoids act as analgesic that reverses any pain and gives the patient instant relief. Some patients have even reported a total elimination of the pain experienced. Studies are replete on cannabis can ease pain. We will look at some of them in chapter five of this book.

Sleep Disorders

Cannabis is known to be able to help patients suffering insomnia. Cannabis can also treat other sleep disorders like having trouble staying asleep, sleeping for short durations and experiencing sleep that is not refreshing. Scientific research into the subject has found that insomnia is a top reason why people use cannabis. Other top reasons are depression, anxiety and pain. A study published in 2019 found that in a group of users who had used cannabis to help sleep, eighty-four percent of them said that they found it very useful or extremely useful. In fact, over-the-counter sleep medicines have been replaced with cannabis by most people when they discovered the potency of cannabis to make sleep more refreshing. Experts see this as a welcome development as they say that a lot of the over-the-counter sleep medicines have been linked to Alzheimer's disease.

The use of cannabis to enhance sleep has a long history that goes back to the seventeenth, eighteenth and nineteenth centuries. Many of these studies show that cannabis can impact on sleep by making you feel so drowsy that it takes less time to fall asleep. Cannabis eliminates insomnia by causing you to feel dizzy almost instantly and in the same manner, it ameliorates different sleep disorders. Experts believe that these effects of cannabis with relation to sleep are tied to the cannabinoid THC. Early studies show that the strains of cannabis that were likely to cause more sleep were THC laden strains. However, another cannabinoid called terpenes also has sleep boosting properties. Terpenes give taste and aroma to the cannabis plant but in addition, it has sedative properties that are good for patients of clinical conditions that cause insomnia. The sedative effects are also good for other sleep disorders and can rectify these immediately thereby relieving the patient of the trouble that accumulates with the inability to sleep.

In recent years, cannabidiol (CBD) has also been found to be capable of inducing sleep. Cannabidiol has gained so much ground in medicinal cannabis that it helps with issues such as anxiety, pain, and even sexual enhancement. Research shows that CBD is affecting sleep also. The cannabinoid is said to be able to improve insomnia symptoms. By causing your body to reach a general place of rest when it deals with other clinical conditions, CBD is helping you fight insomnia and other sleep disorders. Recent research even suggests that CBD may have a more profound effect on sleep than THC.

It is important to emphasize that cannabis can treat insomnia by correcting the clinical conditions that come along with it. A good example of this is comorbid insomnia. This used to be referred to as secondary insomnia. This kind of insomnia arises alongside medical conditions. It could arise as a side effect of medication and other treatments. Research is still underway on this subject and shows that cannabis may be useful for treating comorbid insomnia. Some of the health conditions that can lead to insomnia include physical pain, anxiety, stress and so on. It is apparent through the clinical evidence available that insomnia can be improved once these conditions are improved. In a 2019 study, the data showed that people who used cannabis for insomnia and its comorbid conditions including anxiety, depression and physical pain experienced significant improvements in their sleep patterns and in all the co-occurring conditions. Up to three-quarters of people who participated in that study had at least two co-occurring conditions.

Cannabis can treat sleep disorders occurring with post-traumatic stress disorders (PTSD), intense nightmares, and REM sleep disorder. Because of the range of sleep disorders that cannabis can treat, it is a promising therapy for inducing and sustaining sleep, and research into the area is still active.

CHAPTER FIVE

PROPERTIES AND INTERACTIONS OF CBD IN MEDICINAL CANNABIS

CBD received attention as an important part of cannabis when it was featured in a CNN report by Dr. Sanjay Gupta in 2013. The report "Weed" explored how CBD was used to help symptoms in children with severe seizure disorders. As we have discussed, Cannabidiol or CBD is one of the many cannabinoids present in Cannabis. It is the major constituent of cannabis that is used in medicinal cannabis. This is because unlike THC, it has no psychotrophic effects. Thus, it does not control the moods, emotions or cause intoxication. What CBD contains instead are therapeutic properties and low toxicity that make it useful in medicine. If a person takes too much of CBD, the effects would be drowsiness without any accompanying adverse effects.

CBD tends to be more effective when it is extracted than when it is used in its pure form. The plant extracts contain higher doses of CBD along with other molecules found in the plant extracts. These constituents of the cannabis plant extract all work together to enhance the natural effects of the CBD. Cannabidiol can be consumed in the ways that we have discussed earlier like any other medicinal cannabis. It can be taken orally when it is in oil form and can be used in creams or as a spray. CBD sprays can be used under the tongue. It is not certain what dosage should be used and this can be different from one disease to another. CBD helps to tackle the symptoms of various diseases and offer relief to the patient. Doctors often administer a dosage of 1 mg CBD per kg of body weight and then increase the dosage gradually. The appropriate dosage is then eventually determined.

Topical application of CBD is effective against pain and skin irritations like acne and psoriasis. Most cannabis strains have both THC and CBD components and a lot of them contain these in balanced proportions. In plants like this, the psychoactive effects of THC are lessened and the properties of CBD would be pronounced. If a medication has both THC and CBD, consuming it orally will not reduce the effects of THC. As a result, you have to choose a medication that is specifically designed for medical treatment. Such medication would have the appropriate level of CBD needed to ease the symptoms.

Clinical Conditions That Can Use CBD

CBD and THC are the most researched of all the cannabinoids. Medical practitioners have long discovered that CBD is vital to medical treatments and have researched this cannabinoid extensively. Certain clinical conditions and symptoms have been pointed out that can be relieved with CBD. We will take a look at some of them in this section.

Pain and Inflammation

Cannabidiol has anti-inflammatory properties and analgesic that can be used to fight pain and inflammation. By consuming cannabidiol orally or applying it directly unto the skin, you can ease pain and reduce inflammation. A CBD infused cream can be rubbed on the spot where the pain occurs. CBD has been found to be effective against pain that comes from arthritis.

Antipsychotic Uses

Cannabidiol contains antipsychotic properties that can relieve symptoms of schizophrenia. The use of CBD to aid treatment of psychotic conditions have been widely researched and accepted into medicinal cannabis.

Nausea and Vomitting

A 2011 study shows that cannabidiol contains antiemetic properties that help with nausea and vomiting. The cannabis component is effective against nausea and vomiting that is caused by chemotherapy in particular.

Depression and Anxiety

Cannabidiol is effective for regulating mood and preventing depressive episodes. It is an effective anxiolytic. A 2016 study shows that CBD was effective against anxiety and panic attacks.

Inflammatory Bowel Disease

CBD has been found to be effective against inflammatory bowel disease. It is a useful antidote against conditions such as Crohn's disease and ulcerative colitis. Studies show that cannabidiol reduces intestinal inflammation and inflammatory bowel disease. CBD is therefore essential for relieving these conditions.

Multiple Sclerosis

As with most other medicinal cannabis, CBD and THC are the two active ingredients in Sativex®. The drug is used to treat patients with multiple sclerosis. Another way that the cannabinoid is used is that it is infused into creams that are meant for treating these patients. CBD works effectively to diffuse the symptoms of multiple sclerosis and make the patients feel better. Medical experts have continued to administer CBD infused medication to patients with multiple sclerosis.

Epilepsy

Cannabidiol has been used to treat severe forms of epilepsy effectively. CBD is popular for treating seizures among children who are suffering from epilepsy.

Acne

CBD has anti-inflammatory properties that make it great for treating acne. According to experts, it has a sebostatic effect on human sebocytes. Cannabidiol along with other cannabinoids can effectively treat acne and other skin conditions. They could come in creams that can be applied directly to the affected areas of the skin.

Cancer

CBD has a lot of anti-tumor properties that make it effective in fighting against cancer. Researchers have continued to add to the list of cancer types that CBD can fight. CBD prevents continuous growth of new blood vessel networks that are needed for tumor growth. This anti-angiogenic property of CBD makes it assume an important role in fighting cancer.

Fractures

According to a 2015 study published in the Journal of Bone and Mineral Research, CBD stimulates osteoblast activity that accelerates healing of bone fractures. CBD is thus efficient for correcting fractures.

Diabetes

CBD can both prevent and treat diabetes. It can reduce the occurrence of diabetes and can treat any complications arising from the disease. Examples of such complications are diabetic retinopathy and cardiomyopathy.

Care of the Liver

CBD is capable of protecting the liver from complications caused by alcohol consumption. It can keep the liver safe from hepatic steatosis and any conditions naturally occurring from alcohol or cocaine consumption.

Drug Addiction

Cannabidiol can fight drug addiction. CBD can help you withdraw from cigarette smoking successfully. Similarly, it can aid in reducing opiate addiction.

Neurological and Neuropsychiatric Disorders

Cannabidiol is effective for fighting against neurological diseases as it protects neurons from degeneration.. It can be used to treat Alzheimer's disease among others. It is also effective for fighting against neuropsychiatric disorders.

CLINICAL EVIDENCE OF CANNABIS MEDICINE

In this chapter, we will be taking a look at the clinical trials and peer-reviewed studies that point to the efficiency of cannabis in medicine. Is there real data pointing to the fact that cannabis can relieve symptoms of diseases and effectively treat others? We will be looking at the facts in this chapter of the book.

There are more than 20,000 published studies and reviews that are talking about medicinal cannabis. The use of cannabis in medicine has undergone a more rigorous process of scrutiny than other classes of drugs. Cannabis medicine has to be vigorously checked and subjected to a higher standard than other pharmaceutical products. This is largely due to institutional bullying in the process of getting approval for cannabis medicines.

On the good side, this leads to a large amount of available data on cannabis. There are evidences on cannabis that support its safety for use as a medicine. These legal and regulatory restrictions remain actively operational despite the fact that cannabis has always being in use and has been medically applied to related situations for a very long time. Although its efficacy has different levels of potency from one disease to another, the patients show a strong belief in the ability of cannabis medicine to cure them.

The scientific evidences of the potency of cannabis medicine and the extensive reviews that have been carried out on the subject has made medicinal cannabis available in a lot of countries. Cannabis can now be gotten on prescription in Canada, Germany, Finland, Italy, the Czech Republic, Israel, Spain, Portugal, and the Netherlands. Because cannabis is still restricted at a federal level in the USA, what the doctors can do is offer recommendations. They cannot prescribe cannabis. In the United Kingdom, there are no serious stipulations in place despite that a larger part of the population use cannabis.

Clinical Trials for Medicinal Cannabis in Different Clinical Conditions

Severe Pain

Cannabis is mostly used to ease chronic pain. It is effective for relieving neuropathic pain. Cannabis can cure pain that other forms of strong medicine like opioids and NSAIDS cannot treat. For people who use it along with opiod, they would not need to take a high dose of the later. Cannabinoids are therefore great analgesics. The effects of each type of cannabinoid are different when it is dealing with pain. Patients continue to confirm that cannabis relieves pain long enough to shift their attention from it. In some cases, cannabis can totally eliminate the pain.

There is a lot of clinical evidence to show that it was safe and efficient to treat chronic pain with cannabis. 2007 reports show that cannabis was able to ameliorate neuropathic pain and was an effective alternative to drugs where the patients do not respond to or could not tolerate the drugs. It was also shown in a placebo study that there was a thirty percent reduction in pain when cannabis was used compared to when it was not used in the treatment regimen. This study was documented in the journal of pain that supported the data already available and pointed to the fact that cannabis was effective for fighting pain. In 2008, it was discovered that cannabis was as effective when added to concomitant analgesic therapy as it was when smoked. The Canadian Medical Association Journal reported in 2010 that smoked cannabis could reduce pain, improve mood and help sleep. In 2013, a study showed that cannabinoids were effective for managing pain.

Multiple Sclerosis

This is a clinical condition that continues to benefit widely from the use of cannabis. In fact, multiple sclerosis is one of the first conditions to benefit from medicinal cannabis. It was the first condition for which a medical pill containing cannabis was approved. Research into the use of cannabis to treat multiple sclerosis has focused mainly on individual cannabinoids and there is none pointing to using the cannabis plant as a whole. However, medical practitioners are agreed that cannabis is safe for treating multiple sclerosis.

Cancer

The effectiveness of cannabis for treating cancer is established. Cannabinoids contain properties that fight cancer effectively. The cannabinoids THC, CBD and CBG are particularly effective as anti-cancer agents. The studies on the interactions between cannabinoids and cancer are numerous and there are up to one thousand publications on this issue.

Cannabis is effective for easing the side effects of cancer treatments especially nausea and a lack of appetite. It also regulate mood disorders present in cancer patients including depression, anxiety and insomnia. Cannabis oil has been found to be effective in the treatment and management of many forms of cancer. Doctors are agreed that because cannabis is non-toxic, it has very little harmful effects and is mostly therapeutic. The evidence is tilted towards anti-cancer properties of cannabis in human cell lines and animals rather than its use in treating basal cell carcinoma. Cancer patients continue to find cannabis particularly useful in their treatment regimen.

Clinical trials are still ongoing on the issue of how effective cannabis is for easing cancer pain. Experts are also conducting studies to see how cannabis can help in treating glioma brain cancer.

Alzheimer's Disease

Cannabis has anti-inflammatory and neuroprotective properties that help treat Alzheimer's. The anti-inflammatory properties of cannabis are also helpful for treating a wide range of other diseases such as dementia, autism, schizophrenia, multiple sclerosis, motor neurone disease, Parkinson's disease, AIDS and so on. There is strong clinical evidence to show that regulate, moderate use of cannabis could delay the onset and progression of Alzheimer's disease as well as other neurodegenerative conditions. These studies have been documented in a lot of journals and publications.

Crohn's Disease

Cannabis can be used to treat Crohn's disease, ulcerative colitis and other inflammatory bowel disease. In fact, it has been widely used successfully to treat these conditions. In 2014, a pharmaceutical company known as GW conducted clinical trials that showed that cannabis extracts could treat ulcerative colitis. A lot of people have experienced dramatic improvements in their symptoms shortly after they use cannabis. Some people even report cessation of rectal bleeding. Clinical trials conducted on Crohn's disease patients in recent times have produced astounding results. Up to fifty percent of the patients have experienced complete remission of the disease while more than ninety percent have seen substantial improvement. The clinical trials are well established and the evidence of using cannabis effectively for treating Crohn's disease and other inflammatory bowel disease is conclusive. A 2012 study shows that a treatment regimen with inhaled cannabis improved disease activity index along with other advantages in long standing inflammatory bowel disease patients. In a 2013 clinical trial, cannabis induced remission in fifty percent of patients with long standing Crohn's disease. Similarly, a 2014 study showed that Cannabis sativa was highly effective in treating inflammatory bowel disease.

The clinical evidence shows that cannabis is effective in medicine and is worthy of the place it occupies right now in the medical world. Further clinical studies and research will undoubtedly bring to light more uses for the plant.

CONCLUSION

The thought of using marijuana at all is highly controversial. There are fewer topics that could stir more emotions or arguments than the cannabis plant. The questions range from whether it was safe to whether it should be decriminalized. Policy makers, users, patients and other players are constantly asking what clinical evidence are available and why cannabis should be included in medical treatment. A close look into the topic as we have done in this book shows that the use of cannabis in medicine isn't half as worrying as we all make it seem. Indeed, this shows why there is a surge in its legality across board.

The controversies surrounding cannabis is what led to a research and to continuous study of its constituents. We see that there is more reception according the cannabidiol (CBD) because it does not contain any psychotropic effects. You can as well call CBD cannabis without the high as it is not intoxicating. In this book, we have examined the cannabis plant as a whole and discussed the fact that it has numerous cannabinoids. We have seen that once the high component of cannabis conveyed by THC is removed, the plant and its extracts become extremely useful for treating various symptoms of disease conditions. In some cases, they can significantly reduce or ameliorate the condition itself.

Cannabis has become extremely useful in medicine and the clinical evidence available varies from one disease to the other. As we can see in the last chapter of this book however, the evidence is tilted towards successful use of cannabis in medicine. If you want to be certain about whether or not to include cannabis in your treatment regimen, this book has answered your question extensively.

The issue of the legality of cannabis remains an open question. As we have seen, government regulations in that regard will enhance cannabis research because it will make the plant more accessible and available for the research. Medicinal cannabis has a lot of positive benefits. You have to know how to use it correctly and you have to seek the advice of your doctor before you begin use. This will help you ascertain the appropriate dosage and the method of consumption that you are to adopt. We have discussed the options that you have throughout this book. Once you begin your medicinal cannabis treatment regimen, you can use this book as a reference material to see what you may doing right or wrong. For medical practitioners and everyone looking to explore the field of medicinal cannabis, here is what you need to know packed together in one place.